CCH CONTEMPORARY COMMUNITY HEALTH SERIES

CARE AND PUNISHMENT

The Dilemmas of Prison Medicine

CURTIS PROUT
ROBERT N. ROSS

UNIVERSITY OF PITTSBURGH PRESS

This work is dedicated to
all who suffer from imprisonment—
the inmates and those who must look after them.

Published by the University of Pittsburgh Press, Pittsburgh, Pa., 15260
Copyright © 1988, University of Pittsburgh Press
All rights reserved
Feffer and Simons, Inc., London
Manufactured in the United States of America

Library of Congress Cataloging-in-Publication Data

Prout, Curtis, 1915–
    Care and punishment: the dilemmas of prison medicine / Curtis Prout,
Robert N. Ross.
        p.   cm.—(Contemporary community health series)
    Includes index.
    ISBN 0-8229-3581-3.   ISBN 0-8229-5403-6 (pbk.)
    1. Prisoners—Medical care—United States.   2. Prisoners—Health and
hygiene—United States.   I. Ross, Robert N., 1941– .   II. Title.
III. Series.
HV8843.P77 1988
365′.66—dc19
                                                                87-35331
                                                                CIP

Contents

Foreword

The politician who wishes to survive keeps as much distance as he can from prisons and prisoners. Prisoners do not vote. As a class, they have no influential friends; and the only way they can get attention, short lived as it may be, is by violent actions. No one really likes prisoners, especially the long-term recidivists (repeaters), who are this book's chief concern.

Sometimes it seems that those who know the least about the actual workings and daily lives of the imprisoned are the ones who find it easiest to be experts on prison reform. As governor of Massachusetts, I found an endless supply of people who wanted to tell me what to do.

When I took office in the late 1960s, I inherited the report of a blue ribbon commission which recommended taking the health care of prisoners away from Correction and putting it under the presumably better qualified Department of Public Health. This action sounded good to me. The Commissioner of Public Health successfully sought a grant from the Office of Economic Opportunity (OEO), the so-called Poverty Program, to carry out these changes and I felt we might be approaching a solution to a longstanding source of dissatisfaction.

Much to my surprise, the commissioner selected as director of this project a physician I had known for many years who had a respected position in the academic and medical community, Dr. Curtis Prout. I wanted to work closely with him; but, of course, I could not. Despite my long friendship with him, I thought it best not to intervene, this being a Federal project under a strong commissioner. Prout learned the hard way that the best ideas and best-motivated people can accomplish little without support, money, and above all, power. Now, however, I can take this opportunity to recognize the great frustrations that necessarily came with the job and, as Prout and Ross point out in *Care and Punishment*, were inherent in a plan that was unrealistic and completely unworkable.

In writing this book, Prout and Ross have carefully avoided using such labels as *good*, *bad*, *right*, and *wrong*. Some people may not like this moral neutrality. But for hundreds of years, as they point out, moralizing about prison conditions has not brought about any lasting improvements. The endless, dreary cycle of reform, followed by apathy, neglect, and deterioration, then followed by riots, reappraisal, and reform, will continue until we understand and realistically face the nature of prisoners and prisons.

Prout and Ross show how reasonable standards, enforced by the courts, have made a tremendous difference in many jails and prisons. Prout is a physician with a long association with Harvard University, particularly the Medical School. This book is not a medical text, however. By basing their book on health conditions and medical care, they show that most inmates are different from the general population. They show how very different prison is from any other environment and how devastating this is, not only to the inmates, but also to those who must work there.

Francis W. Sargent
Former Governor, Commonwealth of Massachusetts

Acknowledgments

No book such as this could be—or should be—written without the help and encouragement of many people of diverse interests and backgrounds. Over the decade during which this book was conceived and written, we have benefited from the experiences of many people directly and indirectly involved in the health care of prisoners.

For their generous support, we thank the Charles A. Dana Foundation, the Ella Cabot Lyman Foundation, and the Gardner Family Trust. We thank, too, the staff of the Francis A. Countway Library of Medicine for making available study space and library services.

The superintendents of the various city, county, and state jails and prisons in Massachusetts have been most cooperative as have been the many physicians, nurses, and medical corpsmen. We appreciate the difficulties of their work and hope that our own work has lightened theirs by contributing to the public understanding of the problems they encounter.

Particular thanks go to the staff of the National Commission on Correctional Health Care, especially Drs. B. Jaye Anno and Jay Harness and Messrs. Joseph Rowan and Bernard Harrison.

We have gained particular insights from a visit with Dr. Jack Wright and his staff at H.M. Prison at Grendon Underwood, Buckinghamshire, England.

The Massachusetts Department of Correction has been a valuable source of information. We especially thank Mr. Alfred Di Simone, Director of Health Services.

We have enjoyed working with staff members of the Massachusetts Medical Society, especially Mr. Charles Amorosino and Ms. Susan Webb. The society-sponsored jail health conferences have given us much-needed contact with other workers in the field. Because we participated with them in the accreditation process in Massachusetts, our book has strong roots in the real world.

A few individuals stand out for having made notable contributions to our work and to the field of correctional health—Rena Murtha, R.N., Howard Gill, and Scott Lewis, Esq. The first encouragement to write this book came from Dr. William Bennett, who recognized early that prison medicine is profoundly different from all the other branches of medicine.

Finally, we thank our friends and, even more, we thank our wives, Diane and Trudee, who have tolerated our seemingly endless preoccupation with our subject. Without their forbearance the book would not have been written.

CARE AND PUNISHMENT

Introduction

Before the prison uprisings of the early 1970s, prison medicine was largely a neglected field. Reformers have occasionally recognized that medical conditions in prisons and jails were not what they might be. News accounts have temporarily inflamed popular sympathies for the poorly treated inmates. But, for the most part, the general population has preferred to ignore prison medical care.

After the Attica uprising and riots in several other major prisons in the United States, the inadequacy of medical care became a popular issue. Federal civil rights legislation and interpretations of the Eighth Amendment provided constitutional protection from poor medical care, a form of cruel and unusual punishment. Once the legal apparatus was in place, prisoners and prisoners' rights organizations brought suit against individuals and prisons alleging—and proving—poor medical care. Medical and correctional workers then were forced to examine the unique problems presented by prison medicine.

Attica called attention to the social and political dimensions of medical service. The inmates themselves were not blind to the possibilities of using inadequate health care as one of the justifications for their uprising; although at Attica, as elsewhere, it appears that the riot preceded the stated reasons for it. The prominence given to medical grievances by the Attica inmates once they discovered the political force of the issue made the medical system a burning issue of prison reform.

In response to the publicity, several professional societies, aca-

3

demic institutions, and public agencies began thorough investigations of what lay behind the complaints. They visited some of the clinics, sick calls, dispensaries, and surgeries of the approximately 5,000 jails and prisons in the United States.

After their studies, most of these commissions established standards and regulations. The American Public Health Association (APHA), American Medical Association (AMA), American Nurses Association, American Correctional Association, American Bar Association, and others wrote standards. Later, funded by the Law Enforcement Assistance Administration (LEAA), the AMA began to plan for an ambitious program to visit prisons, evaluate their medical services, and issue certificates of accreditation to institutions meeting the standards.

In the 1970s, at the time the standards and regulations were being written, 95 percent of the inmates of most prisons needed medical attention, two-thirds had never had a medical examination in their lives, more than one-half were drug abusers, and at least 15 percent had diagnosable psychiatric disturbances. Yet two-thirds of the 1,159 jails responding to an American Bar Association survey had only first aid facilities, one-half had a physician who was only on call, and one-third had no physician available.

But adequacy of medical care is a difficult concept. Adequacy is relative, not absolute. People disagree about what constitutes acceptable medical care. The prison population is significantly different from other groups of people receiving medical care. Standards that apply to the general population may not apply as well to the skewed sample of human beings found in prisons. The environment in which prison medicine is practiced differs remarkably from the institutions outside prisons in which medicine is practiced. Importing the value judgments of the outside world to the world within prison walls can do more harm than good.

The most obvious difference between the practice of medicine in and out of correctional institutions is that the needs of prison medicine are subordinated to the higher concerns of security. Outside prisons, access to health care is taken for granted by providers and users of health care. Inside prisons, access to health care and, by implication, health itself are secondary to society's insistence on tight physical security. At Attica, as in so many jails and prisons, a heavy screen separated prisoner-patients from physicians in the examining room. Access to outside hospital facilities is likewise limited by the degree to which outside hospitals can provide secure spaces and are willing to take on the responsibility for the physical restraint of the prisoners under treatment.

The relative importance of *care* and *punishment* in American prisons is one of the major themes of this book. "Offenders do not give up their rights to bodily integrity whether from human or natural causes because they were convicted of a crime. . . . Medical care is, of course, a basic human necessity," according to the National Advisory Commission on Criminal Justice, writing in 1973. "No jail administrator has the right to impose a death sentence, and a failure to provide for the medical needs of those in custody is equivalent to pronouncing a death sentence. . . . The courts leave no doubt that ordinary and decent medical, dental, and general health care must be provided," according to the Pennsylvania County Prisons Standards, written in 1973.

Money has rarely been available for the reform of prison health care; but for a time during the 1970s, emotions ran high enough to make it appear that sufficient funds might be forthcoming. But times have changed since the days of Attica and the popular outrage at poor medical care in the nation's jails and prisons. Social concerns for reform at any price are giving way to more hard-nosed attitudes as the temper of the times shifts.

Perhaps we are better off without the reformer's zeal. Prisons have long been the special domain of the zealot. But, as has so often been the case, when the zealous reformers withdraw their fiery attention from the prisons, so does the rest of society lose interest. There is a high burnout rate and a short institutional memory for prison reform. What we need is a level of emotional commitment somewhere between the exquisite arousal of the zealot and the apathy of the unconcerned.

Despite the flood of government reports about prison medicine, surveys, manuals, news stories, occasional muckraking tracts, and fiction devoted to prison conditions, in almost every country of the world prison health conditions are still deplorable and continue to be denounced. We hope that we are not merely contributing yet another variation on the same old theme—namely, that prisons are terrible places to live in, that no one would live in prison if he had the choice, and that somehow prisons ought to be better than they are. In fact, we have tried to eliminate from this book the "oughts" and "shoulds."

Ambiguity is hard to live with. It is easier to take a clear moral position on one side or another. This may explain why so much thinking and writing about prisons in general and prison health care in particular has been muddled by moralizing. The moralizing may take the "humanitarian" position of deploring the inmate's lot or may take the "authoritarian" position that criminals deserve no better. In either case, however, the deceptively simple and unequivocal moral stance makes it virtually impossible to discern the true ironies and paradoxes of prison medicine, the inherent difficulties of giving the same institution responsibility for both the care and the punishment of its inmates.

Prisons are here to stay. This statement is not an apology for the present correctional system; nor is it a defense. It is a simple statement of fact. It is also a fact that prisons can do serious harm to inmates and to those who look after them. They *are* terrible places in which to live and work; and there seems little likelihood that there will be large-scale improvement in prison conditions in the United States for a long time to come.

What follows in *Care and Punishment* is a series of essays on prison medicine. The subject may seem esoteric; but we hope that our excursion into this limited aspect of the prison problem will teach us something about the larger issues. Prisons are a true reflection of a society's most fundamental values. Beliefs about medical care are likewise based on fundamental values. In looking at the intersection of these two sets of values—the perceived need to punish and the felt obligation to care—we will learn a great deal about both.

Prisons and prison reform are very much in the news these days. Strong feelings have been aroused by attempts to improve the prisoners' welfare. Likewise, powerful fear of the effects of crime, anger at the criminal offender, and desires for revenge have also been mobilized. The cries for "law and order," whatever that phrase might mean, often conflict with the need for justice.

We are not criminologists. We wish we could offer a theory of criminal behavior so cogent that prisons designed according to its lights would be humane institutions capable of reducing the criminal behaviors of the men and women who pass through them. Unfortunately, we must recognize our own intellectual limitations and the limitations of the field called criminology. Post hoc statistical descriptions are useful and important sociological tools but they have not yet produced a reasonable and applicable theory of criminal behavior. Likewise, the fields of medical science, from genetics and molecular biology to psychiatry, have not adequately explained the human impulse to hostile, violent, and assaultive behavior. As a result, partial hypotheses explaining criminal behavior abound. Usually these hypotheses are so ill formed that they cannot be tested by rigorous scientific methods. Perhaps they may never be tested. Science may never be brought to bear on the questions of criminal behavior because controlled human experimentation is anathema—and rightly so.

That leaves us in the United States with severe problems of dealing with a growing prison population, housed in institutions whose proper function and influence are imperfectly understood. We must treat or rehabilitate or merely warehouse men and women who may or may not be predisposed to commit criminal acts. Little wonder, then, that simply *running* prisons and jails has presented great problems.

The great majority of people, who live and work outside prisons, need to understand the unique problems confronting the prison health team. The issues are difficult and emotionally powerful. None is more problematic than the issues raised by providing health care to prison inmates, for practicing prison medicine is not like providing health care in any other setting, including other institutional settings. In his novel *Falconer*, John Cheever describes what happens when an epidemic hits a large long-term prison.

On Friday afternoon, there was this announcement over the PA: "A preventive vaccine for the spread of influenza which has reached epidemic proportions in some cities of the northeast will be administered to rehabilitation facility inmates from the hours of 9:00 to 18:00.

> Wait for your cell call. The inoculation is mandatory and no superstitious or religious scruples will be respected." (p. 197)

One of the prisoners, known as Chicken, voiced a typical reaction.

> "They're trying to use us as guinea pigs. We're being used as guinea pigs. I know all about it. There was a man in here who had laryngitis. They had this new medicine from the needle. They gave it to him two, three days, and they couldn't get him out of here up to the infirmary before he was dead." (p. 197)

In addition to the paranoia that runs rampant in the prison setting, there is the grinding demoralization of the inmates and the people who must care for them. Again, Cheever has caught the tone perfectly in *Falconer*.

> The public address system made [the prison doctor] jump. "Short arm for cell block F in ten minutes. Short arm for cell block F in ten minutes." . . . The doctor, when he was led in, was wearing a full suit and a felt hat. He looked tired and frightened. The nurse was a very ugly man who was called Veronica. . . . The doctor's suit was cheap and stained and so were his tie and vest. Even his eye glasses were soiled. He wore the felt hat to stress the sovereignty of sartorial rule. He, the civilian judge, was crowned with a hat while the penitents were naked with their sins, their genitals, their boastfulness, and their memories exposed. They seemed shameful. "Spread your cheeks," said the doctor. "Wider, wider. Next! Number 73482." (pp. 157–58)

Turning from fiction to the real world, we quote from a letter from Dr. James T. Blodgett, an experienced physician who had been persuaded to take the job of jail physician at the Worcester, Massachusetts, County Jail and House of Correction in 1977. "I thought I could foresee establishing a medical service which would be a credit to Worcester County and an example to all the other penal institutions of the state. Fifteen months later I resigned, frustrated and defeated by the politicians."

Dr. Blodgett went on to describe the inadequate equipment installed in the newly built—but for administrative reasons never used—elegant waiting room, examining rooms, physician's office, and isolation cells of a modern jail infirmary. "With deep regret and the feeling that I wasted a year of my time, I resigned," he wrote.

Another physician who was doing a conscientious job at another county jail in Massachusetts and was very proud of his efforts was quickly embittered by his battle with the accreditation team that visited his jail. He felt that the criticisms of the jail health service were personal criticisms, and he resigned in anger from the Jail Health Committee of the Massachusetts Medical Society and eventually from the Medical Society as well.

It would be depressingly easy to multiply these examples of competent physicians forced, by one means or another, out of the prison health system. To them we could add examples of the many more who remain in the system but who burn out. There are also too many examples of the incompetent physicians who should not have been in any health care system in the first place.

Despite its possibly inflammatory nature, this book is distinctly not a call to arms. Experience has shown that, to be successful in health care delivery, those involved must be nonpartisan. Above all, they must avoid moral judgments. Yet behind our writing of this book, and, we hope, implicit in every line of it, is a profound desire for reform. Merely to develop a workable system of delivering health care in prison and to procure and retain good personnel is, of itself, a profound act of reform. This manner of reform can be carried out without becoming embroiled in the emotional debates of moral, ethical, and legislative issues labeled "prison reform."

Prison medicine is different from all other practices of medicine. We offer here a subjective and objective description of prisoners as people and as patients, the atmosphere in which they live, the people who look after them, the ailments from which they suffer, and the different guises in which these illnesses may appear. The descriptions of the medical problems of inmates in connection with alcohol, drugs, psychological disorders, medical ailments, and surgical emergencies are not intended to represent a complete description of all the ailments associated with prison inmates. In our book, we attempt particularly to show how these ailments and their treatment are different from those found outside the walls of prison.

Jails have iron bars but they also have revolving doors. A report from the Bureau of Justice Statistics shows that 15 percent of released inmates are back in prison within one year, 26 percent within two years, and 32 percent within three years (Jamieson and Flanagan, 1987). In Massachusetts, to give one example, 40 percent of those released with five or more prior confinements were back in jail within one year. These are problems for the "experts" to deal with. But the experts cannot solve these problems without the interest and support of the general population.

There is a large and growing technical literature on criminology, the sociology of prisons, the administration of health care services, and the like (see Jamieson and Flanagan, 1987). The more general treatments of prisons, however, are almost totally lacking. As a result, the public that must ultimately support any proposed changes in prison conditions is left in the dark about the peculiar nature of the prison problem. Yet as criminal behavior and the detention of convicted criminals become increasingly burdensome to society in the United States, there are few general discussions of prison realities. Whether we want to look behind the stone walls and iron bars is not a question any more. We must look. More than 500,000 men and women are now behind bars. The number of prison inmates increased 41 percent between 1978 and 1983, according to a report by the Justice Department Bureau of Justice Statistics. In 1983, there were 8 million admissions to the approximately 3,300 local jails in the United States, an average of 2,400 admissions for each jail.

CARE AND PUNISHMENT

Before the so-called Age of Enlightenment, criminal offenders in the Western world were punished swiftly and physically. The pain and public humiliation were often brutal, but at least the punishment was inflicted speedily. Few prisoners were held to languish in prisons and these usually were not criminal offenders but rather hostages of one kind or another who might be held for ransom or political expediency. Others, not as valuable, were tortured to death, executed, maimed and released as marked men, or simply banished.

With the invention of the penitentiary in Europe and in the United States around the turn of the nineteenth century, physical punishment of offenders assumed a higher purpose—correction of the offender. Moral and religious teaching during long periods of discipline, enforced by the threat of punishment and reinforced by physical means, was expected to remedy the supposed moral deficiencies of criminal offenders and to rehabilitate them for productive lives in society. When the state simply punished the offender's body and assumed little moral responsibility, the societal function of prisons was limited to providing strong physical restraints. Later when the state assumed moral responsibility for months and years of penal correction, prisons assumed the ambiguous function of caring for the criminal offender while necessarily punishing him. Like a firm parent, prison authorities could physically punish the prisoner in the interests of the higher good of strengthening, reforming, or otherwise reaching his soul.

The analogy of the firm parent is an imperfect one, however. Prison officials and guards are not the prisoners' parents. They do not love their charges as parents might. Only in the most abstract sense do prison institutions and personnel *care* for their inmates. In fact, those who do care are often barred from prison work because their emotional involvement with the inmates threatens to upset the correctional system.

Nowhere is this ambiguity more striking than in the case of medical care, for the goals and assumptions of medical care often come into direct conflict with those of correctional policy and discipline. As a result, until recently and with few exceptions, prisons have offered medical care that seemed poor by standards of care outside the prisons. Some jails offered little care; some none at all. Horror stories of poor or absent medical care inside the prisons abound.

Without denying that such horrors might exist, we argue here that the real problems with prison medicine are far more humdrum. The risk of serious health problems in prisons and jails has been relatively low. Prison medicine is dedicated to the treatment of illnesses in a population of people who are seldom seriously ill. In sharp contrast to this day-to-day routine, however, prison medical staffs sometimes must deal with conditions that would tax to the fullest the medical acumen of any physician. These relatively rare medical emergencies are the stuff of which the horror stories are made.

The prison population is young, 95 percent male, and generally healthy. Yet, when given free access to medical attention, as much as 30 percent of the prison population will show up every day for sick call. Utilization of services far outstrips medical need. The complexities of race, poverty, faulty medical care before incarceration, social values, attitudes toward health care and physicians all contribute to the peculiarities of prison medicine. We may add to this the possibility that prisoners are biologically somewhat different from the general population (they are less likely to be hypertensive and more likely to be dyslectic, for example). If such a sizable proportion of the prison population that undervalues medical services overutilizes them, the reasons must be other than medical.

When people think of prisons, if they think about them at all, they are likely to picture jails and prisons as part jungle, part battlefield. This is the view of prison life fostered by fiction, television, and movies because it is the most dramatic. In real life, however, the dominant emotion in prisons is boredom more than fear or rage. Most prisoners are young, strong, and relatively healthy, and they live in cages. Anger got these men into prison in the first place. Prison does nothing to reduce the inmates' level of anger, but sheer survival requires that the inmates hide that anger behind an impassive facade of boredom and alienation.

The Prison Health Project in Massachusetts, directed by Curtis Prout, was a response to the generally felt need to do something about prisoners' rights to health care, dignity, and justice and, indeed, to do something to restore these values to war-torn America at large. A small group of well-intentioned and bright, but otherwise poorly suited, men and women tackled the problems of the Massachusetts prisons. The project failed of its own internal inconsistencies and because of the more general political confusions of the 1970s. A decade later, efforts to reform medical services at Walpole State Prison were rewarded with notable success. This time reform was in the hands of the courts, the legislature, and, somewhat serendipitously, entrepreneurs interested in providing at a profit medical services to the Department of Correction. What the Walpole case may have lacked in reformer's zeal it more than compensated in diligence. There is an important lesson here.

DILEMMAS OF PRISON MEDICINE

There is one spectacular medical problem in jail health notable more for the moral and medical complexity of handling the case than for the large numbers of cases—and that is acquired immune deficiency syndrome (AIDS) and AIDS related complex (ARC). As we will discuss in the chapter on medical disorders, there are no specific "prison diseases." AIDS and ARC cannot be called prison diseases either, although they first came into prominence in the prison population in the New York area. Because several risk factors associated with AIDS are also associated with the prison population (intravenous drug abuse, homosexuality, sexual promiscuity), AIDS is an important disease to prepare for in planning prison health programs.

But there's the rub. How to prepare? The AIDS screening test (whether in or out of prison) is not 100 percent accurate. In a significant proportion of cases, the test will come up positive even though the patient does not have AIDS. What will such a false positive (as it is called) mean in prison? It could be taken as an excuse for isolating the patient so that caring and punitive actions get confused. It could start a panic in the prison. From the point of view of the state, a diagnosis of AIDS can also mean a medical bill of several hundred thousand dollars. And what if the inmate diagnosed as having AIDS is expected to be in jail for only a few more months? Whose responsibility is he? We will discuss these issues throughout *Care and Punishment*.

As Nancy Dubler, a lawyer and professor of Social Medicine at Montefiore Hospital in New York, has written, "In the separated and segregated system designed to infantilize, humiliate, and punish, the need to be cared for is overwhelming." She went on to quote one lifer as saying, "Everything hurts more in prison" (1979, p. 68). As we shall see, when physicians and nurses become more involved in caring, their effectiveness as health care professionals is often diminished or blocked. Society has decided that these people do not deserve caring. Quite the contrary, this function could best be carried out by encouraging, to a far greater degree, visits and associations with outside people who can carry out the caring functions almost in opposition to the custodial and punitive function, thus leaving the medical staff to concentrate on strictly medical matters. It was this conception that split the members of the Prison Health Project and has proven a stumbling block in many other efforts to reform prison health care.

Prison health care is fraught with ethical dilemmas. For example, an inmate is found to have a bullet in his body that is needed by the prosecutors as evidence. Even though this bullet is not a medical hazard and can be safely left in place, should a surgeon accede to the wishes of the prosecution? Can a court order the surgeon to remove the bullet? How can strictly medical values be kept separate from the legal and correctional functions of the jail and prison setting? Finally, how is the quality of medical care to be evaluated in such a setting?

Traditionally, in prison systems medical considerations are subordinated to others. Forensic opinion holds that the bullet can be removed against the wishes of the patient and the attending physician. Professional medical opinion is that the surgeon should take no part in such a decision. Representatives of the American Association of Family Practice and the American Nurses Association said at a recent meeting in Chicago that the health care team should not be involved at all in such a determination.

Another example is the forced examination of body cavities—rectum, vagina, mouth—for evidence of contraband drugs. Most health care professionals involved in prison health work now feel that they should never be required to perform such examinations but that trained correctional personnel should carry out these procedures.

The same applies to the administration of lethal injections for the purpose of legal execution. The case might be made that the physician should administer the lethal dose to make it as humane as possible. However, the practice of administering drugs to bring about the death of a patient directly contradicts the most ancient traditions of the medical profession.

Health education is another aspect of health care that outsiders, at least, are likely to think has application to prison inmates. People are often eager to promote dental hygiene programs and other health education programs in the prisons. It is surprisingly difficult to convince some people that inmates are not especially interested in learning about eating green leafy vegetables or the proper way to massage the gums, let alone the evils of alcohol and drugs.

At the Third National Conference on Correctional Health Care held in Chicago, 1979 (*Proceedings*, p. 52), a group from Michigan reported on their good results in a health education program. They judged their success on the basis of what the participating inmates reported on follow-up questionnaires. Most of the participants reported that they had been "helped" by the education program. Taking the results at face value might give strong encouragement to anyone who would want to set up a similar program. However, before actually establishing such programs in the jails and prisons, these would-be health educators should note that only twenty of the four hundred inmates actually participated in the program. For a group that is bored and will probably do almost anything to escape the tedium of prison life, 5 percent is not an encouraging level of participation.

Finally, there is the dilemma of the medical staff serving in a system they often do not like, treating patients they contemn, for reasons they do not understand, while earning little money or respect either from the prisoner-patients they care for or the correctional system they serve.

A WARNING TO THE READER

This was not an easy book to write and will not be an easy book to read. The emotions aroused by depriving other human beings of rights we hold dear are so powerful they overwhelm rational discourse. The closer one gets to the actual scenes of incarceration, the more horrible the prospect actually is. Prisons are unpleasant places. Paradoxically, however, those people furthest from the actual scenes of incarceration are the most likely to offer an opinion.

Presuppositions, untested assumptions, wishful thinking, and blind repetition of what "might" and "ought" to be are no substitute for the daily struggle to provide health care to a large and growing inmate population. Emotion is often a more comfortable approach to difficult problems than hard thinking. Hard thinking is especially difficult in this context because it seems to lead us into positions already occupied, at least in rhetorical form, by the current economic biases called, for want of a better name, the New Right.

We say at the outset, we do not subscribe to those values and we eschew all political labels. In doing so, we will probably anger everyone a little bit and please no one completely.

The terms *liberal* and *conservative* have lost their meaning and have no place in any consideration of medical care in prisons. Compassion must be channeled toward limited, defined, attainable goals. To be realistic is not to be cold hearted. As it turns out, acceptance of the realities of the situation is the only way progress in prison medicine can be realized.

The clusters of values we have called liberal and conservative shift regularly and as easily as fashion in dress. We have gone through a period in which compassion has held sway. Prisoners' rights had been trammeled in the past; court decisions of the past two decades have restored some of the dignity that remains even when a person is removed from society and put into a prison. Adequate protection of health is surely one of those rights.

We do not believe that good things trickle down automatically from the more favored to the underdog. Nor do we find that those who are unwilling or unable to go to the prisons and jails to work or to listen with an understanding ear to the physicians, nurses, and guards, as well as to the prison inmates, have made any substantial contributions to the welfare of any of them. We do not feel that prison inmates are either good or bad. They are people, out of the mainstream, different, antisocial, alienated—but people nonetheless. There are certain obligations of the state to care for their health and welfare. These obligations can be narrowly defined. To go beyond these limits into moralizing, theorizing, or otherwise to go beyond the ordinary duties of nurse, physician, and corpsman invites confusion.

The tenor of the times, however, now emphasizes other social values. Compassion takes second place to fiscal considerations. Statements of rights are empty promises if public agencies lack the money needed to provide those services guaranteed by right. The problems of the coming decades, unlike those of the previous decades, are thus practical ones. Having affirmed the right to adequate medical attention in prisons and jails throughout the United States, the legislatures, courts, and executive branches of government must now find ways to provide what they have promised.

Looking at the *hows* of a problem leads inevitably to questions of *why*. Every choice entails a ranking of values, for not everything is possible, and every ranking implies a social theory. In the decades of change we have recently experienced, compassion and justice captured the public mind more than dollars and cents. Today public discussion centers on more mundane issues of money but fear and revenge are always on the unspoken agenda. The discussions are nonetheless fraught with passion precisely because between the balance sheets yet another social struggle is being waged.

The time has come for something more than studies and the enforcement of regulations, important as they are. The time has come to understand and deal with the contradictions, paradoxes, conflicting sentiments, economics, and medical necessities of holding more than 500,000 people in American prisons. We need a deeper understanding of the *idea* of caring for the bodies and minds of people we have chosen to punish, rehabilitate, or simply isolate and confine.

Part I
ISSUES AND TRENDS

1

The Cult of Personality
in Prison Reform

HISTORY REPEATS ITSELF

In *Ulysses*, James Joyce has one of his characters offer the opinion that history repeats itself, but always with a difference. The history of prison medicine forces us to the same conclusion. The same controversies concerning quality of care, entitlement to the best available treatment, means of providing the best care, and limited public resources perennially dog efforts to improve the medical service to prison inmates. Strong- and liberal-minded men and women from time to time rise to the occasion and try to reform the system by dint of their prodigious personal powers. But the powers of personal suasion, no matter how great, are almost always inadequate to the task of effecting lasting change in an intractable system. Legends of heroic reformers may persist; but legends are not deeds and good deeds rarely survive the heroes who enact them.

The history of prison reform in Massachusetts has provided two remarkable examples of the temporary successes and long-term failures of the cult of personality. In 1934, Howard Gill, a progressive and effective reformer, the man who designed and ran the Norfolk Prison Colony, was forced to resign his position after politically motivated hearings and a highly publicized public hearing. The Rockefeller Foundation, which had been funding Howard Gill's innovative prison program, threatened to withdraw its annual grant of $55,000 if Gill were forced out of his

21

position at Norfolk. From across the United States, telegrams and letters supporting Gill flooded into the governor's office.

By the time Corrections Commissioner Frederick J. Dillon filed his thirty-six charges against Gill, public interest in the case was at a fever pitch. Commissioner Dillon attacked Gill in the *Boston Globe* (28 February 1934) for what he thought to be "a lack of discipline and an inability to so control the actions of the staff and inmates as is consistent with the proper conduct of a penal institution." When the hearings were begun at the Massachusetts State House, 6 March 1934, the *Boston Globe* (6 March 1934) screamed in a banner headline across page one, "UPROAR AT STATE HOUSE OVER THE GILL HEARING, His Supporters In Near Riot." There were "wild demonstrations of cheering" when the hearing adjourned that afternoon. "Riot broke out" among the five hundred supporters standing in the lobby of the hearing room. Such disorderly conduct was all the more surprising given the nature of the crowd. "The crowd," according to the *Boston Globe* reporter, "contained a large sprinkling of college professors, penologists, and church members."

Perhaps one spontaneous event sums up the conflict of attitudes and beliefs in which the hearings were conducted. As Governor Joseph Ely walked into the chambers, the crowd called him "Caesar," alluding to what they perceived to be the total breach of democratic process in the Gill hearings. Finally, one supporter placed a piece of paper with a crudely drawn swastika on the governor's mantel, with the words, "God save the Commonwealth of Massachusetts." On 30 January 1933, Adolf Hitler ascended to the position of chancellor of the German Reich. In 1934, Hermann Goering made his impassioned speech, "We love Adolf Hitler because we believe deeply and unswervingly that God has sent him to us to save Germany."

For Governor Ely, State Auditor Francis X. Hurley, and Corrections Commissioner Frederick J. Dillon, the Gill affair was mundane politics. "Throughout the latter part of the history," according to one of Gill's staunch supporters, "Norfolk was being jealously looked upon by some of the state politicians, both as a prison where political influence could do nothing for a prisoner, and as a place where jobs were being created and money spent on construction without hope for them or their friends to share in the benefits of either."[1] In a very real sense, liberal-minded citizens of Massachusetts and the United States realized that the moral tenor of a nation can be tested by how it treats its wards, including prison inmates.

In 1948, another nationally recognized liberal prison administrator, Miriam Van Waters, superintendent of the Women's Prison at Framingham, was likewise vilified. Only a massive outcry from the professional and academic community saved her position.

The two cases have much in common; both Gill and Van Waters were progressive, well informed, liberal professionals trying to improve conditions at their institutions. In both cases, the untimely death of a prison inmate sparked public debate over the quality of medical care, but the topic of medical care was really only the wedge by which to open up larger issues of prison governance and still wider issues of how inmates are properly to be treated. In both cases, one of the principal areas of discontent was the medical service. When complaints of coddling the inmates were brought into the open, one of the most common examples of such allegedly excessive leniency was the high quality and high cost of medical service provided to the inmates. In both cases, too, the public took a voyeuristic delight in peering behind the walls; for in both the Van Waters and the Gill cases, there were strong implications of homosexuality and other publicly taboo subjects.

The two cases have yet one more point in common. Both Gill and Van Waters were exonerated and ultimately praised for the proper balance of care and punishment they afforded their inmates. One of Van Waters's supporters described her approach as "the system of individual treatment of those committed to her care . . . in which the forces of science and religion have been fused by humanity into an agency of rehabilitation rather than blind punishment."[2] Howard Gill likewise championed the individual approach to rehabilitating inmates. "As a source of understanding human beings," Gill said, "it seems to me that nothing is more revealing than the man or woman who is without defenses, reduced as it were, to the most elementary qualities of existence."[3]

There may be just a touch of romantic naiveté in the notion that prison existence reduces a person to the "most elementary qualities" so that, given the proper corrective environment, the inmate's character would be strengthened and errors corrected; and that, through humane treatment, inmates would learn to respond as socialized people. As described in a pamphlet about the Norfolk Prison Colony.

> This is the aim of all that goes into the Norfolk plan of individual treatment, the goal of all that is done for and with the inmates. To this end every individual program is constructed; that it may help to dissipate personality conflicts and build character through self-knowledge and emotional catharsis; that by adjusting domestic and social situations on the outside, minor conflicts and unrest may be relieved; that by means of discipline wisely administered, by helpful personal contacts, by discussion clubs, by constructive use of leisure time, and every other influence brought to bear upon him, the man may become an honest, useful citizen.[4]

Sooner or later, however, dissipating personality conflicts, promoting emotional catharsis, relieving minor conflicts and unrest, discussion clubs, and constructive use of leisure time begin to seem— to some people at any rate—more appropriate for the country club than for the prison. "Caring" and "coddling" are all in the eyes of the beholder. Wherever and whenever the the pendulum swings toward conservative and reactionary policies, even the modest minimum of decent care may appear to be pampering.

In summing up the results of "the Norfolk experiment," one sociologist of the time described why the Norfolk experiment was destined to fail.

> The present society does not want such a prison and will not long tolerate it. Whatever penologists may say theoretically about the function of a prison, it is clear that for society in general, it is a place of retributive punishment. The criminal is the scapegoat of society, the whipping boy for all of us. It is easy to appeal to the prejudices of such a society against the "coddling" of criminals in a "country club," particularly when the injustices of that society fall so hard on many of its members who lack even the creature comforts of a decent prison. (Doering, p. 550)

Eventually, Howard Gill and Miriam Van Waters and the reforms they brought to Norfolk and Framingham were swept away
in what one observer has called "the triumph of reaction." We do
not intend to write a history of either the Gill case or the Van
Waters case in the following pages. Interesting as such a narrative
would be, it is not our prime concern to write the biographies of
these fascinating personalities or to chronicle their tumultuous
careers. We are interested in repeating the stories of Howard Gill
and Miriam Van Waters as brief examples of the weaknesses inherent in the reformer's approach to improving health conditions in
the jails and prisons. In succeeding as they did, both Gill and Van
Waters also created their own vulnerabilities.

HOWARD GILL AND THE EXPERIMENT AT THE
NORFOLK PRISON COLONY

At the present time of writing (1987), Howard Gill remains a
charming, bright, energetic, and original man. He is ninety-seven
years old and is still actively interested in prison work. From
1925 to 1946, Howard Gill was involved in various federal jobs
related to prisons and in university teaching jobs. From 1947
until the present, he has been interested in doing research and
teaching in what he describes as clinical criminology. Starting in
1963, Gill taught criminology at American University (Washington, D.C.) and directed the Institute of Correctional Administration. He ran workshops and institutes on various aspects of corrections until as recently as 1980. "They fired me," he said in an
interview, because they had discovered how old he was. At the
time Gill was ninety.

Gill was born in Lockport, New York. A high school teacher
recognized his potential and persuaded him to go to Harvard. In
1913 Gill was graduated from Harvard *cum laude;* the following
year, he was one of the first graduates of the Harvard Business
School. For some time, Gill followed his inclinations in business,
real estate, and teaching at the Harvard Business School. But he
was somewhat undecided as to what to focus his energies upon.

For twelve years, Gill worked with Chambers of Commerce,
both at the local level and at the national level. In his words, "I

either resigned or got fired because my plans were always beyond what the directors thought was possible." Gill ended up, after twelve years, as the National Secretary for the Council for the Prevention of Wars. "At that time, 1926," he recalls, "we were very much concerned with whether the United States should join the League of Nations and the World Court. I couldn't raise enough money for them to keep me so I resigned and I set up an office in Washington with a classmate of mine to look into the competition between prison industries and free industries."

Gill was asked by a group of cotton manufacturers to make a study of the use of inmate labor in running cotton mills, as one way to keep the price down. As a result, Gill spent a year on that subject, visiting all the big prisons in the United States, investigating the question, and assembling the report.

> In those days, a prison warden tried to concentrate on one industry if he could. It was easier that way—either shirts or underwear or furniture or automobile license tags. That didn't sit well with me and I proposed a diversification. That didn't sit well with the cotton garment people. They really wanted to put the prisons into a tight jacket. I learned that they were paying my salary. That's the scheme Mr. Hoover had. He would get some businessmen to put up some money and then they consequently felt they had a special stake in what was produced. And I produced a report which was about to reduce them to a secondary position. They asked me to change it. I said that I could not do that. It would ruin my professional reputation. I told them they could have the report—after all they had paid for it—but that they would have to take my name off it. They considered my proposal for a while. Then Mr. Hoover, who was Secretary of Commerce at the time, gave me five minutes to either change the report or resign. I resigned.

While he was in Washington, however, Gill came to the attention of the Federal Bureau of Prisons, then under the leadership of the great Sanford Bates, formerly head of the Department of Correction in Massachusetts. Bates said, "Don't you change a goddam word of it. You come over and work with me."

Then came the turning point in Gill's career. He was offered the job of superintendent of the new prison being proposed in Massachusetts. Gill took the job on 10 November 1927.

"They had plans for a high-rise, what I call 'medieval, monolithic, monkey-cage monstrosity' and I said so." That became a headline in the local papers. When Gill assumed his responsibilities in November 1927, construction of the prison had been going on for almost six months. By December 1927, Gill had convinced Bates and the Department of Correction to scrap their existing plans. "Bates asked me what I would propose as an alternative. I said, 'I don't know.' They gave me a couple of architects and we came up with a plan in six weeks for what was to become Norfolk, the Norfolk Prison Colony."

The design of Norfolk borrowed heavily from that of the new prison then being built at Lorton, Virginia, in which the customary radial design was replaced by a cluster of individual houses, each with its own living room, dining room, kitchen, and so on. "That seemed a good idea for Norfolk," says Gill. "I proposed a similar design and, to my great amazement, they accepted my plan."

Building the Experiment

The Norfolk Colony is described in a 1932 pamphlet, evidently written by members of the staff, entitled "The New Prison at Norfolk, Massachusetts." The pamphlet is clearly a celebration of the work approaching completion.

> The new prison is located at Norfolk, twenty-three miles from Boston—three miles south of Walpole and the same distance north of Wrentham—very near the main road between Boston and Providence. It occupies a portion of the 1,170 acres of land purchased by the Commonwealth in 1912 for the use of a dipsomaniac [alcoholism] hospital. . . . On the easterly side of this property, several permanent brick buildings were erected for men, and on the westerly side seven wooden buildings were constructed for the women around a circular piece of land called The Oval. The Commissioner of Mental Diseases had supervision of this institution.
>
> It did not prove a success and was finally abandoned, and the buildings remained vacant for several years. After the World War

they were rented for a short time to the Federal Government and were used as a rehabilitation camp for sick and wounded soldiers, and then again abandoned.

In 1926 the easterly part of the property, together with the brick buildings, was transferred to the State Board of Health for a cancer hospital. . . . The rest of the land, including the wooden buildings at The Oval, was transferred in 1927 to the Department of Correction . . . , and on this land the new Prison is built. The original piece transferred to the Prison contained approximately 880 acres, to which has been added 91 acres, making a total of approximately 971 acres.

At the time of construction, the site was actually more a work camp than a prison. On 1 June 1927, twelve men were moved from Charlestown Prison to Norfolk to begin construction of the new prison. Again quoting from the pamphlet of the time,

The first work to be done was to repair, renovate, and make habitable ten old wooden buildings, some of them almost ready to collapse, to be occupied by inmates and officers while the new prison was being built nearby. Small, but well-equipped, plumbing, paint, electrical, and carpenter shops and a very serviceable sewing room were set up in the basements of these buildings. All this was done by the inmates themselves.

There was no wall or fence around the camp, which presented ample opportunity for escape. This was clearly cause for concern, but, in fact, few of the workers took the opportunity. "Of the different inmates lodged here during the period, thirty-five ran or walked away; five came back of their own accord; twenty-three were captured by the guards or other officers; one died; six are still at large."

When the need for a wall became pressing, as it would when the Colony population grew, true to the philosophy of Norfolk, the prisoners themselves built it.

In the construction of the wall and buildings it was decided to use, so far as possible, inmate labor; not only for the sake of economy, but also to teach many men useful trades, so that when they go out they will be better able to earn a respectable living and less likely to resort to those practices which brought them here. Work—hard work—but work in which they are interested and which will be of permanent value to them, is believed to be the best means of making them over into useful citizens.

The experiment has been most successful. Many of the inmates had never done any manual labor—in fact, lack of honest labor, with its attendant temptations, was what brought many of them here. . . .

There has been a vast amount of unskilled labor used in putting in water and sewer pipes, digging foundations and tunnels, laying electric cables, and general grading. Many of the men who could not become skilled workmen did very well in this kind of work. Using the pick and shovel in the open air made some remarkable physical improvements in men who had been for a long time in prison at Charlestown before coming here.

The writer of the pamphlet must have shared, at least implicitly, the faith of the Honorable W. Cameron Forbes in the salutary effects of fresh air and hard work. Forbes was himself experienced in prison administration. He was a former governor general of the Philippines and the initiator there of one of the most advanced penal experiments in the world. He had designed a penal colony in which whole families came to live with the prisoner. Forbes had written in his report after examining the Charlestown, Massachusetts, Prison at the request of Governor Cox, "I came away with a feeling that the inmates had an appearance of unhealthy pallor that spoke of lack of contact with the sun, the great healer of human ills. . . ." Forbes took his muscular Christianity a step further. "Let the sun shine into their faces and I believe some will find its way into their souls" (quoted in Parkhurst, 1939).

The association of work, rigorous exercise, discipline, and strengthened moral fiber was a popular and long-lived one. In 1937, a report of the superintendent of the reformatory at Concord praised military drill by the prisoners. He said, "It is good for their morale" because "it inculcates discipline, with careful attention to physical conditioning, appearance, courtesy, respect for authority, and manliness" (Annual Report of the Superintendent of MCI Concord, 1937). This is almost certainly a reference to the then current notion, dating back to the middle of the nineteenth century at least, that "muscular Christianity" and exercise were good ways to avoid masturbation and homosexuality, those supposed precursors of criminal behavior.

Much later, after Howard Gill was already under suspension from his duties at Norfolk, Governor Ely of Massachusetts, who was hostile to Gill, appointed this same W. Cameron Forbes as the investigator of the situation at Norfolk. Forbes concluded that "Norfolk is the one credible page in the history of prison administration in Massachusetts."

The Gill Case

A simple chronology of the Gill case will help keep the dates and sequence of events in order:

20 April 1927. Commissioner Sanford Bates receives authority from the governor to proceed with construction of Norfolk.

6 September 1927. Twelve prisoners are already in the prison camp and construction of the wall is begun.

10 November 1927. Howard Gill assumes the superintendency.

December 1927. Gill presents to Sanford Bates the proposal to abandon plans for a radial type prison of interior cell blocks in favor of a group of separate buildings after the layout of the Reformatory at Lorton, Virginia. The proposal is approved.

August 1930. A staff physician and assistant are appointed at Norfolk, regular medical service begins three days a week and complete physical examinations of every inmate begin.

1 September 1930. A regular dentist is appointed to work six to ten days per month.

October 1930. The Massachusetts Bureau of Social Hygiene begins research at Norfolk, taking a case work approach to penology.

September 1931. A split develops between administrative and case work groups.

1 October 1931. Gill states the Norfolk policy that in conflicts between institutional needs and the needs of the individual, "the latter must be paramount."

9 March 1932. "Superintendent still insists on prior recognition of the case work attitude. Treatment objectives must not be upset by immediate institutional requirements."

November 1931. Students from Tufts Medical School give complete physical examinations to all inmates.

2 January 1932. Dr. Erickson starts as first full-time resident physician.

13 May 1932. Gill formulates his philosophy of individual treatment.

December 1932. A full-time dentist is appointed.

10 June 1932. Construction of the hospital begins.

1 May 1933. Hospital opens with the transfer of twenty-three tuberculosis patients from the prison camp and hospital at Rutland, Massachusetts.

3 May 1933. The hospital is approved Grade A by the American College of Surgeons.

December 1933. Newspaper coverage begins of the events at Norfolk.

5 April 1934. Governor Ely has commissioner remove Gill as superintendent of Norfolk.

6 April 1934. Commissioner Dillon removes Gill as director of research.

Gill's early triumphs were soon replaced by difficulties. "The fight began three months after I took the job," he said. "The fellow who was behind it all was a fellow who very much wanted to be governor. His name was Francis X. Hurley, the man who proposed to solve all the problems of the Commonwealth with a lottery."

Throughout the autumn of 1933, rumors had circulated about the Gill's leniency and mismanagement of Norfolk. Gill was accused in the *Boston Globe* (9 December 1933) of having allowed Frank Moriarity alias Joyce, one of the inmates, to go "on several hours' honeymoon" after being married at Norfolk. There were also allegations of graft: according to unsubstantiated rumors, guards were forced to pay $280 for their uniforms and equipment, $200 more than they actually cost, "as tribute to higher officials to insure their positions." Gill was accused of altering records when Clarence J. ("Jack") Hapgood and two confederates attempted to tunnel out of Norfolk. An inmate was discovered "1½ miles out of bounds" with a woman. Inmates were said to have made private use of lumber bought for work on the prison. And, according to the allegations against Gill, inmates were allowed to use cameras in the prison and to sell the pictures to the outside.

Gill took the wise course of "pitiless publicity." He opened Norfolk to reporters. By the autumn of 1933, however, as Gill was to declare later in the *Boston Globe* (29 January 1934), the entire case was badly distorted by the politicians, "who were out to get him." The precipitating factor that brought Gill's prison experiment to a close was the discovery of missing funds in the inmates' accounts.

"Howard B. Gill, Superintendent of the Norfolk Prison Colony," was largely responsible for the decision of the Governor [Joseph B. Ely]" to investigate the management of the state prisons, reported the *Boston Globe* (8 December 1933). In November, it was discovered that George Gordon, "an embezzler serving time in the Charlestown Prison," was found to have stolen "several hundred dollars" from the prisoners' accounts. Gill then suggested to R. Clarke Christie, treasurer of Norfolk, that they check accounts at Norfolk. Christie found a shortage of $468—no small amount, considering that a dress shirt cost less than a dollar in 1933 and a new Frigidaire was about $130. Christie, who had been treasurer, was demoted to head bookkeeper and, because he felt responsible for the funds, he reimbursed the account personally. "I am satisfied that the shortage was a result of confusion and errors," said Gill, "and that there was no dishonesty on the part of Christie."

Gill asked for a re-audit, which was begun by the state auditor, Francis X. Hurley. However, in part because a similar shortage had been found in the account at Bridgewater and in part because there had been a recent escape of two inmates from Norfolk, Governor Joseph B. Ely ordered that the investigation be broadened "to investigate all phases of the activities of Massachusetts' correctional institutions. An appropriation was obtained for the purpose. It soon became clear that the investigation was to be confined to Norfolk and rumors appeared that Mr. Gill was slated to go" (Doering, p. 537).

During December 1933 and January 1934, "a series of sensational newspaper stories appeared." There was reason to believe that they may have originated in the offices of the auditor himself.

Then, on 26 January 1934, Hurley "announced that Mr. Gill had been guilty of doctoring prison records in connection with the tunnel attempt of the summer before, and sensational stories appeared in the press making it appear as though the 'doctoring' had been done at the request of a woman, prominent as a Boston liberal, who had sponsored one of the inmates concerned" (Doering, p. 538).

Gill, in his attempt to marshal "the support of an enlightened body of citizenry," had encouraged staff members to speak publicly, as he himself had done, "to support the Norfolk Plan." As a result, the Gill case attracted wide public attention.

Nonetheless, Governor Ely announced that Gill "might be unavailable for the position he had held due to adverse public opinion," and eventually agreed to a hearing to ventilate the Hurley charges. "A number of prominent citizens who had used their influence to secure the hearing, banded together to crystalize public sentiment in favor of Mr. Gill, and above one thousand persons appeared at the State House for the public hearing" (Doering, p. 539), at which the governor "acted as prosecutor, judge, and jury." The hearing lasted four days.

"It was bruited about for some time that the governor would silence the liberals by getting the best penologist in America to take Mr. Gill's post. Several prominent prison administrators were approached but these prospects did not materialize. In the end, the former structural engineer, Mr. Maurice N. Winslow who had been appointed active superintendent when Mr. Gill was 'withdrawn' was made permanent Superintendent" (Doering, p. 540).

Howard Gill remembered the episode in an interview:

I always gave Ely credit for being a gentleman. But he wasn't creative and he had made some foolish remarks. He went on a vacation and when he was met by some newspaper men at the boat in New York asking, "What is going to happen at Norfolk?" he answered, "I'm going to fire Gill." And having said that, he didn't dare change his mind. He was not a bad guy. Senator Parkhurst was interested in prisons. When he learned that I had some new ideas, he hired the most prestigious law firm in Boston, to see that I got a fair hearing when I was charged with 36 allegations of misfeasance and malfeasance. Some of it was true, some exaggerated, some false.

Howard Gill's establishment and operation of the Norfolk Prison Colony and his downfall and removal have a great deal in common with the experience of the Prison Health Project forty years later. In each case, there was a new group of powerfully motivated outsiders, strong support at first from the press and the public, university, and the liberal community. In both instances—that of the Prison Health Project and the tenure of Howard Gill at Norfolk—the support eroded as unrealistic hopes and expectations for reform were unrealized. Criminals were not reformed by Gill's changes, some escaped and accused the prison administration of abusing them, and the issue of medical neglect became the rallying cry and dealt the final blow to reform.

Howard Gill temporarily withdrew 29 January 1934 and permanently withdrew 5 April 1934. His splendid prison physician, Dr. Wilfred Bloomberg, who had just graduated from medical school and who went on to enjoy a distinguish career, resigned when Gill left Norfolk. The new superintendent, Frederick J. Dillon, who took Gill's place, fired the entire nursing staff.

In October 1934, after Gill had left, the American College of Surgeons (predecessor of the Joint Commission on Hospital Accreditation) again accredited the hospital. From this fact we conclude that the hospital was still a good one. Dr. Bloomberg had been replaced by Dr. Louis Sieracki, an internist and recent graduate of Harvard Medical School who was just beginning practice in nearby Norwood.

In the 1937 report of the superintendent of Norfolk Prison, Gill's successor complained that the Department of Correction was not sending him "suitable" inmates. He felt that because of this adverse selection, it was important that custody replace any efforts at rehabilitation. He also pointed out that the previous design of spread-out separate cottages by Howard Gill would make it extremely hard to control a riot. He thought that Norfolk would be appropriate only for the lowest form of security, that is, for what he called the "nice" prisoners. He suggested that the Department of Correction should transfer out the inappropriate prisoners to minimize the risk of riot: in short, "behavior problems, unstable morons, our erratic psychopaths, and all other types of troublemakers" (Annual Report of the Superintendent of MCI Norfolk, 1937).

Health Care and "The Norfolk Hypothesis"

Howard Gill described Norfolk as "the first community prison for men in the United States." It was praised highly by two blue ribbon committees that had examined Gill's work there prior to his trial and removal. He felt at the time that there should be a good prison hospital, staffed by good people, because the added burden of illness, which was not treated, could contribute to delay in rehabilitation. He did not then state, nor does he believe to this day, however, that providing good health will automatically make the inmate more likely to become a good citizen. He still feels, however, that untreated debilitating or painful illness would certainly have an adverse effect on efforts to rehabilitate inmates and that, as a matter of common civil decency, the inmate should be offered a good standard of care.

> One of the first things I did was to go to my boss, Sanford Bates, and ask him to apply to the Rockefeller Foundation for $25,000 to hire treatment personnel. The only people on the official budget were security people. I wanted a whole staff of professionals—psychologists, social workers, educators, and so on. He said OK. I went to New York and they said, 'You don't want $25,000; you want $50,000. They gave me $50,000, $10,000 a year, over five years. In those days, you could get a first-class psychologist for $3,000. I set up a very interesting professional staff of workers. They were the basis of anything I did there that was worthwhile.

E. H. Sutherland, professor of sociology and criminology at the University of Chicago during the height of enthusiasm for the Norfolk experiment, wrote of Norfolk, "This Colony is in many ways the most interesting and promising piece of pioneer work in penology that is being carried on in America." The ideals on which the Norfolk Prison Colony was organized were high indeed.

According to the *Official Manual of the State Prison Colony*, written in the 1930s, inmates were to be guaranteed "a decent routine." "This implies that a man will be given a decent bed, proper clothing, sufficient and wholesome food, plenty of light and air, opportunity for normal recreation and exercise, useful work, reasonable contacts with relatives and friends, through letters and visits, and adequate medical care."

Beyond this "decent routine," the chief goal of the Norfolk Plan, as it was called, was "reduction of criminal tendencies." Inmates were prescribed various routines to promote their "constructive normal development."

> Based upon a diagnosis of the man's needs, a program is outlined for him designed to afford opportunities and help in fulfilling these needs in a normal progressive mode of living. This program is designed to:
>   Increase home and social ties.
>   Increase vocational skills.
>   Increase educational acquirements.
>   Increase avocational skills.
>   Increase recreational interests and abilities.
>   Increase health and physical well-being.
>   Speed maturation through participation in general community activities.

How important did Gill think issues of medical care were? Gill clearly says that he never felt that the medical care was particularly important and certainly had little to do with the *rehabilitation* of prison inmates. Nor did Gill think of medical care as any special right, any more than anything else, his student Yahkub concludes:

> There is no recorded case to show that any one [sic] was cured of his criminality by this new approach of medicine because the forces of rehabilitation on the one hand and recidivism on the other lie fundamentally in the realm of intangibles. They are interlaced and interacting and it is difficult to pull any single string out of the tangled skein. No one could say definitely what particular force produced what particular effect but only guess at the interplay of cause and effect. What one does feel is that the thrust was in the proper direction and that among the contributing causes was the work of the medical division. (Doering, pp. 148–49)

Nevertheless, the Medical Division was an important part of the entire Norfolk plan.

The general health program of the Medical Division for the State Prison Colony is intended to go beyond mere attention to matters of sanitation and attention to cases of definite illness. It seeks to stress the importance of wholesome personal habits and active participation in some forms of outdoor recreation, particularly for those whose vocational placement does not require hard physical labor, and seeks to apply constructive, reparative, medical and surgical treatment to chronic disorders which handicap men both in their vocational and recreational activities.

The Advisory Committee of physicians and surgeons representing the Harvard University School of Public Health determined policies, developed service, and established "wise and proper" methods of handling medical problems. On this advisory board were Dr. Hilbert Day, Dean David Edsall, Dr. Irving Clarke, Dr. Elton Mayo, and Dr. E. B. Wilson.

In a research report dated 27 May 1933, the resident physician at Norfolk in the 1930s, Dr. Bloomberg, maintained,

The Norfolk hypothesis carries the development of medical service one step further along its logical road. All that I have been able to find out about existing medical service in American prisons indicates that in the great majority of cases it is confined to such emergency care of actual illness as amounts to glorified first aid. In line with the program of rehabilitation and attempts to turn each man out better for his stay here, the medical policy has been expanded to include a repairative [sic] or constructive medicine. Of course, the first aid work must be attended to, the general health of the men must be looked after, and the sanitary arrangement and public health features of the Colony must be organized. Beyond these, however, we have the more fundamental problems of constructive work. It includes not only such medicine and surgery as are indicated but also psychological and personal work, close attention to diets, and a program for athletics and recreation.

Just as Norfolk differs from other prisons in its fundamental con-

cept and plan, so it was to be expected that the new prison hospital
would differ from other prison hospitals. Because we are planning
constructive medical work, and because we plan to treat the members
of the Colony as reasonable human beings, deserving of consideration, it was inevitable that our hospital should be more completely
equipped than those of the prisons whose whole aim in its medical
work is to furnish such emergency care as is absolutely necessary.
(Cited in Doering, pp. 226–27)

"It is very difficult to treat adequately a sick patient and at the
same time to lock him up under such a rigid regime." The idea
was to have a hospital that could do everything—everything except maternity, since there were no women prisoners. It was
unusual that the Norfolk medical program was approved by the
Medical Society, even though it had no maternity service. "In
order to do decent medical work," said Dr. Bloomberg, "we must
attract a competent medical staff, and in order to attract a competent staff to our hospital we must meet certain medical standards.
Therefore it is our hope to have the hospital accepted as a class A
institution by the American College of Surgeons" (Doering, p.
227). They were impressed that Norfolk had a first-class program
of training young medical students and nurses and others. Young
surgeons would come out from the Massachusetts General Hospital to do surgery for the princely sum of $100 an operation. Some
of the best surgeons in Boston fought for the privilege of operating at Norfolk.

Norfolk also had a fine medical library. One of the charges
against Gill was that he had bought a medical library with state
funds improperly ("I forget why they thought it was improper,"
says Gill) and sneaked it into the prison at night. It is a sad truth
to report that the same books, of use now only for historians of
medicine, still made up the bulk of the Norfolk medical library
forty years later.

When the prison population was still small, inmates were sent
to local physicians for care as needed. In case of more serious
cases and medical emergencies, inmates were sent to the nearby
hospital. Eventually, Gill found out that one of the inmates was a
physician. "Dr. Silva very foolishly had gotten excited over some

business deals, quite aside from his medical work, and it got him into prison," he recalls. "I liked him very much and I had respect for his medical abilities. When he was paroled, I hired him as my doctor. That was a red flag to the politicians that I would hire my own prisoner—and pay him a salary to boot."

Dr. Silva served as the prison physician quite satisfactorily until two prison inmate deaths occurred. One was a case of pneumonia following a knee injury. "We used to send all our medical cases down to Bridgewater," Gill explains. "But I had a bad experience one time when we sent a man down to Bridgewater. As he was getting into the bus, he stumbled and injured his knee on the wheel. The result was that he got to Bridgewater and died a few days later from some complication. That caused an awful ruckus. I had to prove that I had sent him in a heated ambulance. They accused me of killing him." It may be difficult to recall that, in the 1930s, antibiotics had not yet been developed and medicine was a far simpler art and science than it is today. Deaths that today might easily be avoided, then were more than likely. The two deaths at Norfolk, for example, could not be attributed to mismanagement by Dr. Silva. Nonetheless, the foes of Howard Gill seized upon the opportunity to discredit him and attack the whole operation at Norfolk. Dr. Silva got into further financial difficulties and eventually committed suicide.

Gill did not think there were any struggles with the physicians over sending inmates out because they could offer as good medical care within the Norfolk Prison Colony as could be had anywhere. The hospital had smaller wards than was usual for hospitals in those days—two- and four-bed units, an isolation unit, and the unit for mental patients. An operating room, X-ray, and cardiograph were in the basement, still very much as it is today. Dr. Bloomberg established a convalescent unit in one of the dormitories in keeping with modern hospital practice. This hospital was at the time the equal of any in the country, but standards have changed dramatically since then.

When he started at Norfolk, he said, prisoners with tuberculosis were sent up to the Massachusetts Tuberculosis Sanitarium in Rutland, Massachusetts, outside of Worcester. He got them back to Norfolk and treated them there. Other prisoners were sent down to Bridgewater, where there was a hospital. He would have preferred to have those inmates treated at Norfolk as well.

THE CASE OF MIRIAM VAN WATERS AT FRAMINGHAM WOMEN'S PRISON

A seemingly endless supply of prison reformers has not exempted Massachusetts from recurring charges of inadequate prison health care. The only explanation can be the extraordinary ability of people and of institutions to forget the unpleasant and the insoluble problems so often associated with prisons.

Women's prisons have many of the same problems as men's prisons in this regard despite the usually greater expenditures and outside support for women's prisons. In the mid-nineteenth century, the great Dorothea Dix toured the country exposing to the public the terrible conditions in the prisons and jails of the United States. Her great influence was felt locally in the charter for the Massachusetts Women's Prison in 1876. In what would appear now to be a forward-looking move, the charter called for a full-time registered nurse, a resident physician, and for mandatory physical examinations of the women inmates. Among the early superintendents of the Massachusetts Women's Prison was Clara Barton.

In the 1930s, Dr. Miriam Van Waters, a national figure in criminology, was lured from California to Massachusetts and set about vigorously in many directions to make of the women's prison at Framingham a humane and rehabilitative institution. Her roster of medical advisers and consultants in the 1940s was a veritable Who's Who of leaders in Massachusetts medicine, gynecology, obstetrics, and pediatrics. Almost all had or later attained professorial rank at Harvard and Tufts University Medical Schools.

Dr. Van Waters, too, was subject to attacks increasingly as a "coddler" and "an apostle of permissiveness" who, by lack of public condemnation of homosexuality, was accused by implication of encouraging it among her women inmates. Again, the charge of inadequate medical care was the lever used against her. The fulcrum was the post–World War II ground swell of public sentiment against liberal reform in prisons. The suicide of a young female inmate, allegedly the lover of a young female staff member, was presented as prima facie evidence of bad care. A sensational and vehement collection of charges against Van Waters led to her complete vindication after a strongly vocal outcry from the educational, medical, and liberal political communities.

Within twenty years of Dr. Van Water's retirement, the medical care at the Framingham Women's Prison was again condemned for its failures to provide adequate medical care.

THE MORAL OF THE STORY

Strong individuals make a difference for a while but, like all heroes, they pass away. Their influence may continue for a time, but, more likely, they have already created their own antithesis. The major problem with the cult of personality is that it invites personalized, and therefore emotional and bitter, attacks. What is needed, instead, is a more enduring, more businesslike, more institutional control of prisons and jails.

A single person or a small interested group, regardless of how powerfully and right-minded, cannot create enduring changes. The dedicated prison physician burns out. The overworked and undersupported nurses, the mainstays of any prison health system, quit. The socially motivated public action group moves on to the next hot social issue. Legislators forget. The print media sell newspapers and the electronic media sell broadcast time by moving on to other stories of the minute.

2
The Prison Health Project

Few people would deny that providing good health care in prisons and jails is a problem. Furthermore, most people would agree that if rational people work hard to define the problems and to propose reasonable solutions to them, sooner or later at least partial solutions of the problems would be forthcoming. This has not been the case. In the best of all possible worlds, reason might prevail. In the imperfect and confused world we actually inhabit, reason is only one of the contending forces.

There are many important unresolved issues concerning the health of prison inmates. The question has been how to deal with them. Reasonable people do not always understand the problems. They expect limited and provisional solutions to remedy systemic problems, or they propose global and ill-specified solutions to particular and limited problems. At the same time, less rational colleagues and fellow citizens often act as if reason is not the chief means of dealing with prison problems. Emotion—both sympathetic and antipathetic to the plight of the prisoner—clouds the issues and prevents their satisfactory resolution.

Power in the United States is divided among three branches: the legislative (regulations and finances), the executive (action and implementation), and the judiciary (prosecution, conviction, precedents, and standards). The Prison Health Project had some of the power of the executive, but only that. The case of the Prison Health Project shows the inability of the executive branch, no matter how powerful, to achieve its goals without the support of the other two. Nine years later, armed with a set of national standards established in part earlier by the Prison Health Project, the judiciary, by court order, and the legislature, by grudgingly appropriating more money, enabled the executive to carry out many of the original objectives.

Each person has his or her own ideas of justice, the nature of prisons and prisoners, and society's true wishes. It is in the nature of things, as we shall see, that humane, cost-effective, and cost-beneficial medical care of acceptable quality is possible in correctional institutions but only by sharpening the focus on particular programs, lowering global expectations, and establishing a sound organizational structure within the correctional system itself.

If we can learn from our mistakes, the story of the Prison Health Project in Massachusetts from 1972 to 1974 is a powerful primer. It is the story of a group of supposedly intelligent, hardworking, strongly motivated people trying to carry out a seemingly reasonable plan based on seemingly reasonable assumptions. The charge to the Prison Health Project had its genesis in prisoners' demands that sounded not only reasonable but also practicable. The reasons for what was and was not accomplished are complex and will appear only as we look in greater depth at the nature of prisons and prisoners and the health care delivery problems peculiar to prisons. Idealistic goals proved to be no match for the hard facts of life.

Following the uprising in the maximum-security state prison at Attica, New York, inmates in the maximum-security prison at Walpole, Massachusetts, virtually seized control of their own prison. After several days of violence and negotiations, inmates of neighboring Norfolk State Prison issued their demands for better health care. Soon after, inmates of Walpole issued a similar set of demands. As at Attica, improved medical care was a major demand, medical care being a more tangible and more appealing rallying cry to the public than "justice."

Among the demands were the following:

1. Twenty-four hour care must be available with a registered nurse on duty.
2. Medical emergencies must get more attention and reaction time to emergencies must be shorter.

3. Inmate nurses must get medical training.
4. Prison physicians must have full medical authority in diagnosis and treatment.
5. Prison physicians must have the authority to order rest and relief from the daily routine (lay-in time).
6. Medications given to prisoners in pill form must not be crushed but rather must be given whole.
7. Every prisoner must get a complete medical examination on admission and periodic examinations as needed after that.
8. Prisoners in segregation units must be visited every day by the physician doing rounds.
9. Prisoners must have access to private consultations with physicians outside the prison system as needed.
10. Medical specialist visits to prisons must be increased.
11. Programs of dental therapy must be improved and expanded.
12. Inmates must receive training in dental therapy.[1]

Innocuous or inscrutable as these demands might appear to the uninitiated, they nevertheless posed almost insurmountable problems when tested by the realities of prison medicine. As an introduction to the sometimes baffling complexities of prison medicine, we will discuss each of these seemingly innocent demands.

Twenty-four-hour care with a registered nurse on duty is an accepted idea, but, under the existing laws, labor shortages, and limited funding, staffing these additional positions was impossible. Even if the money for their salaries had been forthcoming, the difficulties of recruiting the nurses would have answered the inmates with a resounding no.

More efficient management of medical emergencies, likewise, is only a humane and reasonable request. Nevertheless, the inevitable demands of security placed barriers of time and space between the accident victim and eventual definitive treatment.

Medical training for inmate nurses, a liberal, high-minded, and seemingly reasonable notion, in practice became the subject of manipulation, contrary to the provisions of security, and failing to lead to positive certification. In no place where such training has been tried has it succeeded or been continued.

Dispensing pills intact, and not crushed, as the inmates had complained of, seemed an innocent enough demand. In fact, however, inmates often have a thriving trade in pills of all sorts, garnered from sick line and traded or sold in the active drug traffic that exists in just about every prison. Inmates learn very quickly that they can feign taking the pill, holding it in their cheek pouch until they are out of sight of the nurses, and then retrieve it for sale. Crushing the most actively sought pills, naturally, makes this practice impossible and interrupts the drug traffic.

The remaining demands—proper medical examinations on admission to the prison, daily rounds to segregated units, increased dental and specialist care—were all desirable improvements in prison medical care but difficult to realize under the constraints existing at that time and still existing in most places.

THE MADOFF COMMITTEE

In response to the worsening situation in the state prisons in Massachusetts, the secretary of the executive Office of Human Services appointed a study committee drawn from various fields of health (principally public health), penology, and consumer affairs. Morton Madoff, director of the Division of Laboratories in the Department of Public Health, convened the Medical Advisory Committee on State Prisons. Twenty-three medical, dental, public health, and community representatives first met in October 1971, at the request of Peter C. Goldmark, secretary of human services, and John Fitzpatrick, commissioner of correction. Although many members of the "Madoff Committee" had had some experience in delivering care in various institutions, they had very little experience in providing services in prisons. None had worked as a prison physician. According to the Madoff Report,

> Inmates of each institution presented a cataloguing [sic] of specific grievances, with cited instances of alleged medical neglect, at least the general nature of which were confirmed in many instances by corrections officers and other personnel, including those responsible for health care delivery. The committee, however, has chosen not to present these anecdotal observations in the report, although it is prepared to document the foundations on which its observations are

based. The committee is concerned with the factors influencing the basic quality of care in prisons, and with the recommendation of those changes necessary to bring this care to an optimal level, regardless of the antecedent quality or the specifications on which the determinations of the level of that quality were founded. Unfortunate instances of poor medical care have undoubtedly occurred in our penal institutions in the past. Some will certainly happen in the future. The committee hopes that its recommendations, when carried out, will help to minimize the frequency of these and that all persons, employees, and the public, as well as inmates, will enjoy an improved sense of security concerning the health environment in the penal institutions in Massachusetts. (p. 2)

It is well worth examining the intentions and assumptions of the Madoff Committee, as reflected in their report. (1) The inmates' allegations of "medical neglect" were accepted as the working assumption of the committee when, in fact, they should have been investigated as the research problem. Although the committee rejected as "anecdotal" the inmates' reports of negligence, they then dignified the anecdotes by calling them "the foundations on which its observations are based." (2) Correction officers, other personnel, and "those responsible for health care delivery" are suitably vague sources of information. (3) The committee announced that it wanted to take a more abstracted view of the "factors influencing the basic quality of care" and would "bring this care to an optimal level." The intentions of the committee, likewise, may be laudable but are difficult to define with any precision. (4) Finally, the committee made recommendations without showing how they might be carried out to give employees, inmates, and the general public "an improved sense of security concerning the health environment in the penal institutions in Massachusetts."

At its initial meeting, in consultation with Commissioner Fitzpatrick, the Madoff Committee decided that "any meaningful response to the prisoners' health concerns would require an analysis well beyond a mere investigation of the specific items put forth by the inmates" (Madoff Report, p. 1). Interestingly enough, however, in compiling its report the commission spent almost no time at all in actually talking with anyone who had served as a prison physician.

The assumptions of the Madoff Committee are worth close scrutiny, for at the outset the report (pp. 1–3) asserted that its work was "rooted in certain basic assumptions concerning the role of health care in correctional institutions."

> First of all, while the Commonwealth may be obligated to exercise its protective and rehabilitative role by committing convicted criminals to institutions, it must be careful not to subject the prison inmate to special risks to health or life. Basic health rights should not be denied to prison inmates any more than to other members of our society.

The second assumption of the Madoff Committee concerned the intrinsic rehabilitative power of good medical attention—a thesis that has yet to be supported by fact.

> If an inmate is confident that his health needs will be met, he is more likely to make a positive adjustment to the institution's affirmative programs. Fear of inadequate medical attention is an important part of the prevalent sense of alienation and deprivation in our correctional institutions.

Third, the Madoff Committee assumed that the commonwealth takes on the role of guardian when it imprisons a convicted criminal. In that role, the commonwealth is obligated to provide the best medical care available, even when that level of care greatly exceeds the level of care normally sought by the inmates in their civilian lives.

> When imprisoned, the inmate loses the right to choose. His health care becomes the responsibility of the Commonwealth and the correctional system, and the prisoner should be afforded access to as qualified a level of care as he might desire to seek out were he not institutionalized. The State, moreover, has the opportunity to improve the level of health and the health awareness of this disadvantaged segment of society. A quality system of health care is an integral part of a meaningful rehabilitative program.

Finally, there is the definition of health itself. In this, the Madoff Committee members took, in their own words, "the broadest conception."

> Health care must concern itself with those organic, emotional, and behavioral qualities which contribute to an individual's antisocial and criminal behavior. Not to deal adequately with these issues is to resign ourselves to the continued staggering social and financial costs of our present system's failures.

The Madoff Committee adopted an essentially medical model by which to understand the social, psychological, and correctional status of the inmates. Prisoners, in the words of the report, "have an unusual burden of unmet health and emotional needs, which are compounded by the unusual stresses of prison life." Consequently, "we are concerned about the health care of inmates because we do not believe that they, as human beings, have forfeited the right to compassionate and individual care."

We see here, already, the mixture of advocacy, moralizing, and criminology reflecting the confusion in the minds of this admirable committee as well as in the general public of the real goals of prison health care. We also see the common tendency of medical and nonmedical people alike to attempt to transfer and apply the methods and goals of medical science to problems that may have little to do, directly, with medicine.

There is now no disagreement that providing adequate health care is an obligation of those federal, state, and local authorities who put some citizens into prisons. The United States Supreme Court and lower courts throughout the country have reinforced the notion that prison inmates have a rightful claim to adequate medical attention and that to neglect the medical care of inmates is to infringe on the constitutional prohibition of cruel and unusual punishment.

We are left to wonder, however, whether the obligation to exercise "its protective and rehabilitative role" entails other special obligations. Again, in the words of the report, an inmate's "positive adjustment to the institution's affirmative programs" seems, in some way, to be tied directly to medical care. The "prevalent sense of alienation and deprivation," for example, is attributed, in large part, to the "fear of inadequate medical attention." A "meaningful rehabilitative program" thus requires "a quality system of health care."

This argument is implicit in the Madoff Committee's definition of health itself. A function of medical care, according to the committee, is to remedy "those organic, emotional, and behavioral qualities which contribute to an individual's antisocial and criminal behavior." Prisoners are human beings. Human beings deserve better treatment than to suffer untreated in prisons. Inmates have not "forfeited the right to compassionate and individual care." These are minimum requirements of any humane system. But there remains the question of what constitutes that optimal level of care. Is it the best the state can provide with its available funds? Is it the level to which the inmates were accustomed before they were imprisoned? Is it, as the committee concluded, that level of care the inmate "might desire to seek out were he not institutionalized"—or even, as Dr. Jay Harness of Michigan maintains, the best care that can be offered? What are the positive benefits of even the best medical attention? Is it legitimate to expect that the best possible health care "is an integral part of a meaningful rehabilitative program"? Why?

The Madoff Report was a creature of its age, and it is more than a purely intellectual exercise to examine the assumptions of this fascinating document. The assumptions of the intelligent and well-intentioned people who comprised the Madoff Committee are the assumptions of most well-intentioned people who become even marginally involved with prison health care. The problem is that the assumptions rarely get tested by reality. It is easy to *feel* that something must be done about prison health care. It is likewise easy to *say* that something must be done to improve prison health care and easier yet to find fault with those whose efforts have fallen short of the ideal. It is extremely difficult, as anyone who has spent an appreciable amount of time trying will attest, actually to *do* anything to improve prison health care.

The Madoff Committee published its findings in late December 1971. A "proper health care program," according to the report, "must seek to detect and repair existing defects, maintain a high level of health during incarceration and, insofar as possible, prepare the convicted offender to cope in a normal manner with society when he returns to it." To accomplish this goal, the Madoff Committee proposed sixty-eight recommendations for improving general medical care, dental health, nursing, occupational and environmental health, training, rehabilitation, and such participatory programs as in-prison medical experimentation and blood donations programs.

This use of the medical model for the identification and treatment of deviant behavior and social adjustment rests on several assumptions. It is an assumption that in a prison setting any serious rehabilitation program can be carried out capable of helping an inmate "cope in a normal manner" with the free world when he returns to it. Even if such long-term rehabilitation were possible, it is an assumption that one could get properly trained psychiatrists, psychologists, and social workers to work full-time in the prison to make a difference.

Perhaps the most important part of the Madoff Committee's report is the two-sentence conclusion (p. 49):

> The Committee finds that there is no clear line of responsibility for the delivery of health services or for the supervision of the health environment in the Massachusetts correctional institutions. We feel that much of the failure to deliver adequate health care is directly due to this lack of coherent administration in this area.

This diffusion of responsibility—one might even say evasion of responsibility—may well prove to be an unconscious or even deliberate act of aggression against prisoners. Prison administrators are unwilling to make medical decisions "in an area in which they have no technical expertise." Medical personnel, on the other hand, are "uncertain of the limits of their responsibility and of their relationship with the correctional aspects of the institutions and are left to work out these problems almost entirely on an ad hoc basis."

Again, in the words of the Madoff Report,

> The quality of medical care is thus compromised. Medical personnel tend to become involved in consideration of custodial and disciplinary

needs rather than in the advancement of health care. Work habits are frequently shoddy, disciplined administration of health care services is lacking in most cases or, at best, is well below the standards maintained by those responsible for the problems of custodial care.

The criticism was correct but, as is often the case in such committee reports, blames the victims (in this case, the health care team) for the inadequacies of the institutions within which they work.

The principal recommendation of the Madoff Committee for realizing these goals was the establishment of a separate Division of Prison Medicine, independent of the Department of Correction and under the supervision of the Department of Public Health. This plan to reform prison medicine was not surprising. The city of New York and the federal prison system had made similar changes. But even at the time of the Madoff Report, serious problems with the arrangement were becoming apparent. The federal government had increased the role of the Federal Bureau of Prisons while decreasing the role of the Public Health Service. This change in federal policy, needless to say, shifted the locus of control to corrections rather than health and welfare, a shift that was rarely acknowledged.

In September 1972, Massachusetts had a new commissioner of public health. Dr. William Bicknell was a young, liberal-thinking physician from the OEO. The regulars of the Department of Public Health thought he was a bit of a wild man, but he had been picked by Governor Sargent from the OEO Health Services particularly for his ability to shake up the long entrenched civil servants of the department. For the most part, they were conservative, cautious, underutilized, and afraid of change. Each year, the Department of Public Health cared for fewer and fewer patients in its public health hospitals and clinics. Tuberculosis, the traditional major raison d'être of Public Health, was coming under control. The hospitals for tuberculosis, chronic alcoholism, and mental illness were being phased out by "deinstitutionalization." Thus the Department of Public Health was becoming a department without a mission. The Madoff Report promised to give the Department of Public Health a renewed mission.

FORMATION OF THE PRISON HEALTH PROJECT

The Madoff Committee and the Departments of Correction, Public Health, and Human Services hired Jane Katz, a consultant from California recruited for her special expertise in getting grants from the Office of Economic Opportunity (OEO), popularly known as the "poverty program." The OEO was established by John F. Kennedy and abolished by President Nixon after the 1972 elections. Bicknell and Katz submitted a proposal for a model demonstration project to carry out the goals described in the Madoff Report. The proposal was accepted, and in mid-1972, a nonprofit, nongovernmental grantee known as the Massachusetts Health Research Institute (HRI) was authorized to accept funds for the Massachusetts Department of Public Health. HRI announced that it had received a one-year $336,000 grant from the OEO to improve prison health services and to develop a model narcotics addict rehabilitation program for prisoners. The money was to be divided into $250,000 for prison health services and training programs and $86,000 for a model program for the rehabilitation of narcotics addicts to be housed at the old Shirley Industrial Home for Boys.

Political, social, and personal antipathies surrounded the Prison Health Project as Governor Sargent accepted the task of implementing social reforms proposed by the previous administration. The political environment was supercharged. Sargent was the Republican spokesman for the Camelot associated with the Kennedy years; Attorney General Quinn was the defender of the Democratic Boston political establishment. Throw into this internecine strife Goldmark, a bright, young, liberal Jew from New York, and Commissioner of Correction Boone, an outspoken black also from outside Massachusetts. By the time the grant was announced, Corrections and Human Services had already picked out most of the personnel, leaving the incoming director little latitude. The day Dr. Curtis Prout started work on the Prison Health Project, the Boston *Globe* ran the headline story that Attorney General Quinn was about to recommend to Governor Sargent that he fire Secretary of Human Services Goldmark and Commissioner of Correction Boone. Quinn had lost the gubernatorial election to Sargent and took upon himself the role of vocal opposition.

An important feature of all OEO activities was consumer participation. In this case, the consumers of prison health services were the inmates, so they were required by law to participate in the planning and implementation of the OEO-funded program.

These features of the contract were put in place before the director was appointed. The director of the drug rehabilitation portion of the project was a forty-five-year-old man who had been in and out of prisons since the age of ten. Some time before being appointed to direct the drug rehabilitation program, he had decided to go straight while serving a term for heroin addiction in a hospital for the criminally insane. He was an invaluable source of information about the realities of prison life, the forces at work, and the habits of the prisoners. It is not surprising, however, that he did not have highly developed organizational skills.

Another requirement of the contract was that a medical advisory council be set up in each of the state prisons. Meetings were to be held in the prisons for the convenience of the inmates, who were to comprise at least half of each health committee. The other members were strong advocates of the prisoners' rights and wants. It is not surprising that the minutes of these committee meetings, dutifully circulated to the members of the Departments of Correction and Public Health, were heavy on rhetoric and reflected the wishes of the prisoners. Inasmuch as there was no power, money, or mandate behind them, however, these reports of prisoners' demands and wishes had little or no effect other than to allow the inmates and their advocates a platform from which to state their heartfelt and usually very real grievances.

The immediate objectives of the Prison Health grant were simple to define before the project actually got under way. Once the realities of the situation became known, the objectives and means of achieving them became infinitely more complicated. In the innocence of first formulation, the objectives were to recruit more health services staff to work in each of the four state prisons; develop improved procedures for comprehensive health care delivery in the prison facilities and between prison and civilian health delivery systems in a cooperative effort by the medical community, inmate health councils, and staff of the Department of Correction; establish health careers training programs for inmates and develop employment opportunities for trained inmates on their release.

These charges of the grant were unrealistically broad. No one in the federal or state system gave the Prison Health Project any guidance, power, or legal support in implementing such a broad mandate. Worse yet, the project contract prohibited the use of funds for operating or implementing programs. Although the avowed purpose of the grant was to plan only, the project members and the prisoners and the state officials expected the Prison Health Project to take definitive action and to pay for services to the inmates. With several different constituencies represented in the project, the proper course of action to take was often unclear. But the members of the project were expected to devote their energies and limited resources simultaneously to divergent areas of concern.

Perhaps the easiest goal was to develop a model health care system for the state prisons that could be used in other states and possibly for the federal prison system. The planning was relatively straightforward. The project's plan, soon drawn up, had a table of organization, lines of responsibility, job descriptions, emergency plans, and medical practice standards. Others had made such plans before, recently in New York City and San Francisco. On paper, plans are foolproof. In practice, there are always problems.

The second goal was to develop and implement programs for training inmates in various medical and paramedical fields and to find job opportunities for them after release from prison. We shall see how in the real world of prisons the objectives ran directly counter to the paramount concerns of security.

The third goal was to assess the drug problems in state prisons, describe treatment programs, and make recommendations for implementing such programs. Enthusiastic, educated liberals, motivated by the best of intentions but without police powers or special training, were ill equipped to discover the basic facts of drug use, distribution, and power politics within the prisons. Inmates and corrections officials each had a well-developed agenda. The unseasoned investigators were caught between the powerful demands of inmates and officials and were no match for either group.

The fourth goal was to establish jointly with the Department of Correction a Narcotic Rehabilitation Project at the abandoned Youth Services Correctional Facility in rural, isolated Shirley, Massachusetts. Since this project preceded the overwhelming national use of drugs, there was little reliable information on how to proceed with a rehabilitation program. Fifteen years and billions of dollars later, the goals, methods, and results are still unclear, although one can see the errors of the past being repeated in the present.

Amid overwhelming needs and demands from inmates and correctional workers for direct support, money, supplies, and personnel, the Prison Health Project was, by its various mandates, increasingly constrained by the contractual agreement to do no more than produce research findings. By definition, the research results were to be measurable, predictable, and reproducible. Numbers, quality control, and accountability become key issues in a milieu that, in many ways, prohibited attention to such "academic" details. On the other hand, attempts at assuring justice were forbidden by the terms of the contract. In response to the rhetorical demands of the inmates, many of the public, news media, and staff of the project itself felt compelled to redress some of the wrongs they saw.

The Prison Health Project began in September 1972 with four staff members: Dr. Curtis Prout, director; Richard W. Clapp, deputy director; Margaret "Sunny" Robinson, director of training and placement; and Helene Lyne, administrative assistant. The contract was signed in early September 1972 but the money did not come through for another two months. In the meantime, Prout had to lend some members of the staff money to live on. Commissioner Bicknell provided for a few small offices in the old building then being used by the Department of Public Health at 600 Washington Street in Boston, but the project staff was excited and optimistic.

The first weeks of the Prison Health Project were devoted to becoming familiar with the setting. An agreement of understanding was signed during this time by the Masssachusetts Departments of Correction and Public Health, the Office of Human Services, and the Division of Youth Services to "jointly share responsibility" for the medical care of adults and juvenile offenders. The specifics were not written, a politically wise but administratively disastrous omission. Power and control remained outside the project.

Director Prout was the oldest of the group. He was a practicing internist whose administrative experience had been confined to a well-structured and well-financed university health service, where he had worked in the painful process of developing a clear delineation of responsibilities and powers. He had in fact learned a good deal about the perils of entering into an unstructured organization in which the lines of responsibility were deliberately left blurred.

The deputy director, Richard W. Clapp, was the son of a pediatrician. Clapp had been a medical student at Columbia College of Physicians and Surgeons but dropped out. Disillusioned with the medical establishment, Clapp took a degree in public health, worked under the Division of Health and Hospitals in New York City, where Frank Rundles and others were revising the New York City Prison Health Care System under Health and Hospitals, directed by Leona Baumgartner.

Sunny Robinson was a nurse-educator from Columbus, Ohio. She was an ardent radical, a crusader for women's rights, a champion of justice and liberty. To the end, she felt that the principal purpose of the Prison Health Project was to enter the eternal struggle for justice, liberty, and equal rights. In the long run, she led a revolt of the project staff and Prout had no choice but to fire her, which caused five more of the staff to quit. The chief disagreement, of which Robinson was the most vocal spokesperson, was over relationships between the Prison Health Project and the "establishment." For Robinson, emotion overrode policy, the ends justified the means, and compromise was anathema. She was bright, warm, and personally compelling, radiating a sense of power and determination.

Helene Lyne was a more mature woman, literate, warm, and intelligent, whose blend of liberalism and realism was a welcome antidote in the heady atmosphere of radical reform. She was the first to express the fact openly that the diffuse mission and global goals of the Prison Health Project were counterproductive and bound to fall short of expectations.

The project secretaries themselves reflected the biases of the project. One was a highly disadvantaged and very appealing man who needed the money desperately but who was hopelessly incompetent and soon was let go. Another was an angry crusader who could not accept her role as secretary. Yet another was an inmate, out on work furlough, who was one of the most likeable members of the project and certainly one of the most "laid back." Her secretarial skills were minimal but her skills at manipulating the system were great. It was hard not to like her but difficult to see where she could be of use.

The director of the drug rehabilitation portion of the project had spent considerable time behind bars between the ages of ten and forty. He was streetwise, tough, humorous, likeable, and appropriately skeptical that we would produce anything of lasting benefit. His ideas of how to reform the long-term recidivist criminal were startlingly realistic. For example, one day in a relaxed social atmosphere outside of the project, he said to Prout, "You know, Doc, all this business about rehabilitation and training social workers and other reformers in the prison is a waste of time." When pressed for his solution, he said that, after many years of first-hand observation, he had concluded that by some unknown process, some recidivist criminals were going to make it and some were not. He felt that somewhere between the ages of forty and fifty, a good number of them, himself as an example, decided to kick the habit of antisocial behavior and go straight. He felt that this came about by being repeatedly hurt when society exacted its revenge or punishment. He said, in effect, that if any therapy worked, it would be group therapy among peers.

When Prout asked him how he would manage the long-term inmates in Concord and Walpole, he came up with an idea, perhaps original with him, but certainly one that is not mentioned in the literature of criminology. He maintained that any person with spirit and a modicum of brains, with twenty-four hours a day to consider his imprisonment, would see the prison walls as a challenge. He suggested that we take the drug rehabilitation project in rural Shirley, with its housing and dormitories surrounded by no walls in sight. In the woods, if necessary, there could be several walls encircling the compound. But these would be out of sight of the prisoners so as not to be a constant reminder and challenge. He would then give each prisoner a certain amount of money to feed and clothe himself and to attend to his wants for the year. He would then say to the inmate, "Here's where you are going to live for the next few years. Here's the money. Take care of yourself. If you mess up too badly, you will spend the rest of your life in solitary or in a maximum-security prison." Those who got the message and behaved would be let out and would become, he expected, useful citizens.

The trainer and coordinator of prison medics was a Viet Nam veteran, warm, witty, sharply antiestablishment. His experience and skills as a trainer, as well as his organizational expertise, lagged behind his likeable qualities.

The two nurse trainers on the project worked with tact and gentle persistence. They were probably as effective as anyone on the project in their attempts to develop programs, record statistics, and make life a bit easier for the nurses in the prison medical system.

These formed the core of the project. Around them, from time to time, were various consultants and other workers, each with his and her own biases, strengths, feelings of commitment to bringing about change.

Inevitably, the tolerant attitude of the director in his refusal to fire several of the activists, despite repeated demands from various quarters to do so, led to a demand from Washington, as well as from cabinet-level people in Massachusetts, that a hard-nosed administrator be appointed. This was essentially a prerequisite for continuing the contract. The man who was appointed was indeed what had been asked for, and he was the direct antithesis of all the people then in the project. He neither needed nor courted popularity. He studied every last paragraph, sentence, and word of the contracts and orders, which most of the rest of the project personnel had skimmed over or neglected entirely. Likewise, he insisted that, in the work of the project itself, every *i* be dotted and every *t* be crossed. He perceived from the beginning that liberty, justice, and loving care might have their place, but not within the confines of the Prison Health Project contract. It was only a matter of time before he came into direct conflict with the rest of the project staff.

To learn firsthand about the prison situation, nearly every day one project staff member or another visited the four state prisons for long-term convicted felons and the large state hospital for the criminally insane. All are within a relatively short commuting distance of the city of Boston, in the eastern part of the state.

The maximum-security prison at Walpole, having a capacity of 500 and an actual population of inmates ranging from 500 to 700, had been notorious, as a source of trouble from the day it opened. Allegedly it was built in a hurry during the Depression, using, for the sake of speed and economy, plans that had been paid for by the Federal Bureau of Prisons but soon abandoned as unworkable.

Within shouting distance, but divided by a town line, is the Norfolk Prison designed and first run by Howard Gill (see chapter 1). Norfolk is slight larger, also maximum-security, with a somewhat less awesome reputation and somewhat less frightening group of inmates than Walpole. Built in 1930, its hospital, the only one in the state prison system, was once the model for the country and a training ground for young surgeons and other physicians from the Massachusetts General and other great teaching hospitals of Boston. Norfolk had fallen on very hard times, however, by the time the Prison Health Project began.

In Framingham was the only women's prison, with an original capacity of more than 500 but at the time of the project having about 100 women and within the next few years housing 30 to 50 men as well. It is not a maximum-security institution and escapes were not rare.

In nearby Concord is the other maximum-security institution, with a somewhat less fierce reputation than Walpole or even Norfolk. But in its appearance, its overcrowding, and the polarization between angry inmates and the officials, it is just as formidable as the other institutions. More of the inmates at Concord were, at that time, incarcerated for drug charges and, by an unspoken design, Concord had the largest percentage of black inmates and the greatest degree of racial polarization. Prout attended one of the meetings sponsored by the Jaycees at Concord, where virtually the entire white population attended and not one of the blacks.

MCI Bridgewater was the most remote and physically isolated of the institutions under the Department of Correction. Not only did it house the so-called criminally insane, but also it housed the Treatment Center for the Sexually Dangerous Offender and a large unit for disturbed chronic alcoholics. Bridgewater was never visited by the original Madoff Committee, was never mentioned in the Prison Health Project contract, and was the object of neglect by many members of the Department of Correction. The staff at Bridgewater felt, quite rightly, that they were being ignored. When the Prison Health Project did pay attention to Bridgewater, the staff members there were almost pathetically grateful. Ironically, despite its poor image and isolation from the rest of the correctional system, Bridgewater was the best-run institution of the five. This is probably because of the work of a dedicated and tough-minded administrator who directed the facility.

There were three minimum-security forestry camps, which the Prison Health Project staff visited at least once. The numbers of prisoners were very small, security minimal, and the problems of health care not at all pressing compared to those in the larger institutions.

The fourteen county jails in Massachusetts were not a charge of the project, but ten were conscientiously visited. The other four adamantly refused to allow visits by the project staff.

The project people, working on a small federal planning grant with no state titles, power, or pay, had on their side only the power of persuasion and a tiny amount of money. At the top was Governor Francis Sargent, a highly personable, public-spirited, and liberal Republican—in a state with 70 percent Democratic registration and a small splinter of Republicans, many of whom were more liberal than most of the Democrats. Sargent came to office at the wrong time in history for him, as President Nixon and the conservatives were rapidly gaining control of the national

Republican party. As a result, Sargent had no political base either at home in Massachusetts or in the national party.

Sargent had appointed as secretary of human services Peter Goldmark, an intellectual and a global thinker who made no effort to ingratiate himself with the Massachusetts politicians. Under him at first as commissioner of corrections was John Boone, a liberal black who came from the federal system. He too had an almost invisible political base in Massachusetts. William Bicknell, commissioner of public health, was the person who had put the OEO grant through and had intended to house in his department a division of correctional health care. Bicknell was also an outsider, neither part of nor sympathetic to the Massachusetts political fellowship. Nor was he sympathetic to either the powerful Boston academic medical community or the established medical society. The dislike was mutual.

At one time, Bicknell's department had run twelve large hospitals throughout the state, in an era when tuberculosis and chronic alcoholism were public health responsibilities. There had been a large number of experienced clinicians dealing with these serious clinical problems. With tuberculosis no longer a disease to be treated in isolated hospitals for long periods and chronic alcoholics being deinstitutionalized, the large hospitals had very little function. On paper, this was an ideal opportunity to match the medically underserved prison system with the dramatically underutilized public health system. This design, incidentally, pleased neither and turned out to be completely unworkable. The only tangible liaison worked out was the establishment and opening of a maximum-security ward in the Shattuck Hospital, bellwether of the state's public health care system.

During the time of the Prison Health Project, the Massachusetts Department of Public Health had 4,500 employees, a new hospital, and a large new division of laboratories in nearby Boston.

THE PRISON HEALTH PROJECT—ALL THINGS TO ALL PEOPLE

The difference between staff and line functions is always a concern of any organization. In departments of correction, this gap seems to be especially sharp; everyone would like to get away from the line. Few people prosper in the day-in, day-out confinement within prison walls under unpleasant and unsettling circumstances. Moving to the central office is more comfortable, more socially acceptable, and is usually associated with a promotion. This gap was especially deep in Massachusetts at the time of the Prison Health Project; but the project served to make it even more pronounced. The administrators who were to "share jointly" in responsibility felt that the project belonged to them and was created to do their bidding. The beleaguered workers in the prisons, welcoming any bridge to the central office and hoping for attention and money, counted on the project for support.

The Prison Health Project was expected to fill a vacuum. Prout's understanding when he took on the project was that he would be director of "special health care programs" under the Massachusetts Department of Public Health and director of the prison health grant administered by the Massachusetts Health Research Institute. Having no clear set of objectives and no written guidelines, Prout tried to do everything: keep the guards happy, practice medicine, plan programs, take on administrative details, and do the necessary politicking to keep all the many factions of the Prison Health Project, the correctional establishment, and inmates working together.

The needs were greater than any single agency could satisfy. More important, as the demands on staff and directors of the Prison Health Project became increasingly diverse, the regulations by the OEO became increasingly severe and restrictive. As a result, the Prison Health Project was expected to do all things for all people when, in fact, it could do very little for any of them.

As director of the project, Prout had an abrupt introduction to the realities of the situation. On the first Sunday morning of the existence of the project, after the newspaper releases, Prout was called from church to Walpole.

"Why are you calling me?" he asked on the telephone.

"You're the doctor," was the quick reply.

"I'm not your doctor," said Prout. "I'm a planner."

"OK. But there isn't any doctor and this man has a knife in his chest. What am I going to do?"

Naturally, Prout drove out to Walpole. Thus began his painful dual role as planner and physician, an introduction to the fact that he would not be a desk-bound planner making pronouncements but rather was going to be the first line of defense against growing disorder in the Massachusetts jails and prisons.

Shortly thereafter, Prout had the point reinforced when an acting medic at Walpole called Prout to say that there was no physician on call at the prison and Prout should come immediately to examine an inmate who was complaining of severe chest pains. The man had been known to have a bad heart; and so Prout had little choice but go.

On his way out to Walpole, Prout thought that the trip was an annoyance but, in any event, he would be able to get on with the rest of his rounds as soon as he had examined the inmate. In his naiveté, Prout thought that practicing medicine in the prison setting would be like any other practice. No. Once Prout was at the prison, medics and inmates quickly realized that they had access to a physician and paraded an endless series of complaints before Prout. In three hours, Prout saw twenty-eight people with a variety of disorders: abdominal pain, herpes of the ear, hepatitis, finger fracture, infected eye, abcess of the buttocks, and, as always, insomnia, indigestion, and the late results of beatings and injuries, the history of which was never revealed.

Medical records were in disarray. Early in the Prison Health Project, a surgery consultant ordered elective plastic surgery for an inmate at Norfolk. One of the state psychiatrists countermanded the order, saying that there was no need for corrective surgery because there was no significant disfigurement. The inmate remained adamant. The issue was eventually referred to the Prison Health Project, but there was no record of decisions in the case. In trying to document the history of a patient's complaints, the workers in the Prison Health Project often found that records were lost, orders conflicted with each other, and the names of the consulting and attending medical staff were illegible or missing entirely.

Throughout the project, petty concerns took on the gravity of profound ones:

- In June 1974, a Quaker woman sharply questioned the project director about the treatment of violent women, saying that any prison for women was a sexist institutional attack on all women and must be abolished.

- The Deputy Commissioner of Public Health proposed getting uniforms for the medics. "They look sloppy without uniforms," she said. In a program that could not find money for beds and medical supplies, salaries for competent nurses and physicians, requests for uniforms bordered on the ludicrous. More outrageous still, this same Department of Public Health probably had hundreds of uniforms stored away somewhere but would not volunteer any for the project.
- The Peaceful Movement Group, a concerned citizens' committee, called the Prison Health Project to say that they wanted to have their own doctors posted inside correctional institutions to monitor the quality of care. When the Peaceful Movement Group was encouraged to send physicians, none appeared.

On 18 September 1972, Prout had his first meeting with the Lifers' Committee at Walpole. He was led into a bare room behind the chapel. Gradually, before the meeting came to order, the guards disappeared and, soon after, so did the assistant superintendent. Prout was left alone with the fifteen angry, verbal, and unyielding inmates. The meeting lasted two hours in the hot and airless room. The sheer exhaustion that followed that session culminated in a night of insomnia. The encounter spoke volumes, however, about the effect on prison health personnel of daily exposure to such a barrage. Physicians are generally accustomed to being asked hard questions, but the satisfaction of being able to do something usually eases the burden of answering difficult questions. In this case, the questions were unanswerable and the solutions were beyond the powers of the project.

"Where is Jimmy Lightfoot's hand cream?"

"Why was there no medic here yesterday?"

"Duncan wants regular Fiorinal for his headache."

"Bobby Delillo wants a transfer."

"Why are guards handing out the medicines when they are not competent medical experts?"

"Why do the guards crush the pills before they give them to us?"

"Can the medics be paid more than 50 cents a day?"

"Why has it taken nine months to get Bruce Manley across the street to be treated at Pondville Hospital?"

Bobby Delillo was eventually transported to Pondville Hospital for the X-rays he had so violently demanded. He appeared in his cloth examining gown, with a gun, and made his escape. It was later learned that the "gun" had been carved from a bar of soap and had been painted with shoe polish. The likeness was good enough, however, for Delillo to use it to disarm the guards, march them to the van, take one of their uniforms, have himself driven to a wooded reservation not far from the hospital, handcuff the men to a tree, and make good his escape.

Men with nothing to do but think about how to outsmart the correctional and medical authorities are, not surprisingly, often quite successful. Patients feign angina and emphysema, hoping to be transferred to more desirable facilities. Other inmates complain of a bad heart and hyperventilate to be relieved of work details. A prisoner pulled what turns out to be a fairly common trick of swallowing a razor blade wrapped in waxed paper. The paper does not show up on X-ray but the razor blade lodged in the patient's esophagus appears with alarming clarity. Prison-wise physicians watched the patient but did nothing. The blade passed and no surgery was needed. Less-experienced and skeptical physicians, on the other hand, were easy prey for the con games concocted by bright, imaginative, and angry inmates.

For a long time, professional members of the Prison Health Project staff conscientiously paid attention to every complaint and allegation. Often they repeated the errors of the Madoff Committee, who accepted the reports of the inmates at face value. As one inmate said to Prout, "These people aren't called cons for nothing."

In June of 1973, Prout received the first of many calls from a young prisoner at Norfolk, complaining of severe and dangerous abdominal pain, "which they don't pay no attention to," he said, "and nobody cares." Attending to his complaint within twenty-four hours, Prout learned that this man had appeared at the sick-line five days a week, month in and month out. Five years later, long after the project's demise, Prout received a call from an inmates' advocacy committee in Boston asking him to investigate the terrible act of injustice being committed against this same man in Norfolk Prison.

In the outside world, such patients are treated symptomatically. Nothing can be done about the underlying personality disorders driving their hypochondria. In the prison, where character disorders are commonplace, the hypochondria takes on a kind of normalcy and is treated with more dignity than it receives in the outside world.

Nor are the guards always exactly as they appear. At one of the first meetings of physicians, medics, correctional officers, and project members in October 1972, a big guard, well known to the inmates and project staff, complained about allegations that guards were smuggling drugs to the prisoners. "I'd like to get my hands on anyone who says that. Listen," he said, "we're there to help them." A month later, this guard was found with a bottle of 200 Nembutal capsules.

The early days and weeks of the Prison Health Project were a very shaking experience for Prout and to varying degrees for the others involved. Separating the realities of the difficult medical situation from the inmates' manipulations of the situation for their own advantage proved difficult and even impossible at times. The intention to do good would not be enough to guide the Prison Health Project through these troubled waters.

EARLY DAYS OF THE PRISON HEALTH PROJECT

In a search for tertiary care centers to provide medical services to inmates with the most severe medical problems, Prout explored the possibilities afforded by the Department of Public Health. At that time, the Department of Public Health had 4,500 employees, general hospitals in Boston and Springfield, and chronic disease hospitals—Pondville, Lakeville, Tewksbury, Rutland Heights, Massachusetts Hospital School in Canton. Most of these were old tuberculosis hospitals and, in 1972, were woefully underutilized since tuberculosis was no longer the scourge it had been.

Until the successful establishment of the maximum-security unit in the Lemuel Shattuck Hospital, the Department of Correction had taken care of all patients at the prison hospital in Norfolk. The more serious cases of bad wounds, severe fractures, head injuries, and like had been sent to the Boston City Hospital or to the nearby Norwood Hospital. The city of Boston, always in dire financial straits, was owed well over $1 million by the Department of Correction, and the physicians at the Norwood Hospital were hard pressed to take care of the flow of inmates to their emergency room in 1972 and 1973. They tried to refuse them altogether on the grounds that it disrupted the treatment of regular patients at the hospital. The solution was political and almost brutal. The Norwood Hospital at that time was applying to the State Public Health Council for a Certificate of Need to build an addition. The Public Health Council, presided over by the commissioner, made it clear that a certificate of need implied obligations to the public which, in this case, included the care of prisoners. Hard feelings created by this action remained a problem for years.

The first tangible solution to the emergency problem, there being no adequate medical or surgical staff or equipment to take care of illnesses or injuries in the prison system, was for the project to forge an agreement among the five largest medical school teaching hospitals in the Boston area. The plan was for the several medical school hospitals to take the serious emergencies in rotation. The load on any one institution was not onerous, about half-a-dozen cases a month. This solution worked well for many years, in part because each hospital knew that the others were also carrying a share of the load.

Financing medical care was one of the serious problems. During the first month of the project, it occurred to the project staff that the most obvious solution was to have Medicaid fund the care of inmates. This program, massively funded by the federal government, was designed to insure adequate medical care for the indigent. Certainly prison inmates satisfied that criterion; but the attitude of the public toward convicts deliberately excluded prisoners from coverage.

Prout's efforts to find reasons for this block and to get anyone in high office to take on the fight for Medicaid coverage of inmates, logical as it seemed, continued without success throughout the duration of the project and for many years thereafter. The diffusion of power and responsibility among the local, state, and federal agencies proved an ideal mechanism for evading responsibility with a clear conscience.

Staffing was another major problem for the Prison Health Project. Prout tried to get Dr. James Carolan, formerly the prison doctor at Norfolk, to return to prison medicine. Carolan was a capable and conscientious physician who been severely criticized by the Madoff Committee report and felt that he had not been given an opportunity to explain to them what he knew about the realities of the situation. In fact, although the Madoff Committee had interviewed inmates, guards, officers, and outsiders, they never interviewed the man in charge of medical services at Norfolk. Carolan politely but firmly declined Prout's invitation.

Prout then turned to three extremely capable friends of his, highly regarded internists in the town of Walpole, near two of the major prisons. Prout wrote to each of them, appealing personally and on behalf of the Medical Society for help in providing prison medical care at Walpole. The primary duties of the physician would be attending sick call and carrying out physical examinations. The pay for this full-time job was $25,000. Not surprisingly, not one of the three responded to the offer.

Looking further, Prout talked with the local head of Selective Service about releasing conscientious objector physicians to work in the prisons. The physician draft was still in operation in the early 1970s. Work in the prisons would therefore have been an acceptable alternative to military service. Major Griffiths, the man in charge of the program, replied that it was an interesting idea but that he had no drafted physicians at the moment nor did he have any conscientious objectors at the moment whom he could divert to prison work. After this disclaimer, the major concluded, "But if I can be of any help, just let me know."

From time to time, physicians would offer to help. Sometimes they were responding to ads in the newspapers or professional journals; sometimes they would simply volunteer. One was a well-qualified internist who was a Quaker and peace activist. He had not been at Walpole for more than a few hours before he fled in tears, leaving word that he would never return.

On another occasion, a board-certified neuropsychiatrist applied to work in the prisons. This sounded too good to be true. Indeed on investigation, it appeared that he had been committed to the Bridgewater State Hospital for sexually abusing his patients. His license to practice had been suspended.

Another bright, personable, and energetic physician who was completing his training for certification in emergency medicine was hired by the project but, as it turned out, he was also drawing a full salary from the Commonwealth of Massachusetts for being a prison health administrator and moonlighting in the emergency room while also getting another half-time salary from one of the major teaching hospitals in Boston. He was endlessly imaginative in finding shortcuts. When he was cut down to merely one or two salaries, he left.

When the Prison Health Project started, the physician at Norfolk was Richard DellaPenna. He was extraordinarily devoted, able, and intelligent. DellaPenna had been recruited in 1972 from his residency on the Harvard service of the Boston City Hospital to help at the time of crisis when there were no physicians to serve at Norfolk. DellaPenna and his colleagues at Norfolk accomplished prodigious changes within the limits of budget and personnel. When there was no physician at Walpole, DellaPenna even took on those responsibilities.

DellaPenna maintained that there should be a state division of prison medicine based at Norfolk Hospital and not run by administrators in Boston. He had been led to believe that the Prison Health Project was to give him direct support in personnel and money to carry out this plan. Needless to say, this confusion of expectations led to disappointment and eventually to irreparable breaches between the project staff and DellaPenna.

DellaPenna's base of support in the Department of Correction was divided. The Department of Public Health was not forthcoming with the support that they had led DellaPenna to believe they would deliver. As a result, angry telephone calls, memoranda, and meetings failed to lead to any workable arrangements for solving the problems between Norfolk, Walpole, and Boston.

To heighten the confusion between the responsibilities of the Departments of Correction and Public Health, there was the newly created Executive Office of Human Services, based on the federal HEW model. This superagency impinged on prison health care.

All this was happening at the height of deinstitutionalization of mental hospital patients and chronic alcoholics. With no other place for these people to go, more and more of them ended up in the jails and prisons. Task forces and special assistants from the Office of Human Services visited the prisons, setting up programs in drug rehabilitation and alcoholism. Among them there were many experts aware of the shortcomings of others but remarkably few who would accept responsibility or do the line work.

Simple things turned out to be virtually impossible. Walpole, for example, needed partitions and curtains to afford some degree of privacy to patients being examined. Equipment and furniture for the clinics and emergency rooms were hard to find at the prison and were beyond the scope of the budget. Even the most rudimentary articles of equipment and supplies were too expensive to buy or simply got lost in the bureaucratic tangles of requisitions and orders.

Meanwhile, the Massachusetts Civil Defense and National Guard had a gigantic warehouse in Natick, where were stored surplus supplies from World War I and World War II. While half the cells in Walpole Prison had no mattresses or blankets, this warehouse held under armed guard at least a thousand mattresses moldering into uselessness. More important, perfectly usable, if somewhat antiquated, X-ray machines were in storage, along with sheets, bandages, cooking utensils, blankets, cots, and more. Despite this embarrassment of riches, even the twelve stretchers Prout requested would have stayed in the warehouse gathering dust if Prout had not gone on a foraging trip with the governor's wife. By enlisting her sympathy and energy, the project got a few items from a grudging bureaucracy, but earned some new enemies in the state system.

Money was short throughout the system. Everyone in the state was concerned about the deficit and the politicians were unwilling to raise taxes. They expected the project to perform many of the state's functions.

One solution was for the state not to pay its obligations. At the time, the Commonwealth Department of Correction owed Boston City Hospital over $1 million and Massachusetts General Hospital more than $600,000. Correction officials said that they would not pay these bills because Boston City Hospital and the prisons were both state-supported institutions. Why, they argued, should they simply transfer money from one account to another? Why they would not pay the Massachusetts General Hospital, however, was another question. Eventually the MGH refused to keep any longer a man sent there with multiple bullet wounds in his chest. When Prout told the people at MGH that Norfolk did not have the capacity to care for the patient, he was informed that the inmate's bill was approaching $100,000 and that the state had no intention of paying. The inmate would have to go. With luck and hard work, the man eventually recovered in the Norfolk Prison Hospital.

PASTORELLO AND DELLAPENNA

This was the necessary background for the emergence of a tough, realistic, pragmatic man who wanted to work at Walpole Prison instead of talk about it. Prout had placed a small advertisement in the *New England Journal of Medicine*, describing in general terms the need for a full-time physician at Walpole Prison. This journal has the widest readership for a medical journal in the English-speaking world, but the advertisement attracted only two responses.

The first was from a woman physician who wanted to know why they published advertisement referred to the prospective physician as "he." Prout admitted that the reason was that he expected no woman physician to be interested in the job but that she was welcome to apply. She persisted in abusing Prout for offending the women physicians but eventually hung up without volunteering herself or her colleagues for the job.

The other response was from Dr. Ernest Pastorello. Pastorello appeared in Prout's office toward the end of October 1972. He had been a highly respected general practitioner in Milford, Massachusetts, and an extraordinarily hard worker. After an illness, he was forced to slow down. When he presented himself to Prout, he was looking for a new challenge. He did not ask Prout many questions in that first interview. Rather, he took one look at Walpole and said that he would take the job with one stipulation. "If you can get the prison hospital cleaned up," he said, "I will be able to run it."

Dr. Ernest Pastorello stayed on the job for more than two years, surmounting all sorts of obstacles. He seemed to thrive on the fight and reached an accommodation with DellaPenna and the neighboring Norfolk Hospital. He began to work on the details of getting the medical facilities in order. In this he had little support from the man who was at the time superintendent of Walpole, an irascible man named Vinzant. Vinzant was a disciplinarian who had been brought in from the outside as the dictator to bring order out of chaos. Rumor had it that Vinzant's hero was General George Patton and, indeed, Vinzant did carry a pearl-handled pistol.

In any event, the prison was hardly large enough for both Vinzant and Pastorello. But when Vinzant left, for he did not last long on the job, Pastorello persevered and soon won the complete support of DellaPenna and the superintendents of both Norfolk and Walpole.

DellaPenna at Norfolk and Pastorello at Walpole supplemented and supported each other and between them made remarkable progress in restoring Walpole to order. Pastorello trained his medics, established the previously disordered record system, and even succeeded to a large degree in removing the inmates, particularly the Prisoners' Rights Union, from their position of strength within the Walpole infirmary unit. Prior to his coming, the prisoners' rights organization decided who would get to see the doctor and even attempted, on some occasions, by threats or intimidation, to decide what treatment the inmate should receive. More than once Prout had experienced these attempts at intimidation when taking the sick line.

Until the prison was brought under control by the security forces, it was impossible even for Dr. Pastorello to set up a completely workable system. In retrospect, it is hard to believe what things were like at that time. The door to the infirmary wing was open a good deal of the time and even when it was closed, the bars made it possible for a large group of inmates standing in the corridor to observe just what went on in the sick bay. These people, known to the medical staff as "gate hangers," shouted their own words of advice and encouragement and were a constant nuisance and even a menace.

It became immediately apparent to the project that privacy was a major problem at Walpole. It was agreed on paper by the correctional authorities, the prison authorities, the physicians, the medics, and in fact anyone who was part of the situation, that the simple matter of putting a steel plate over the open gate and removing the entrance to the more easily defended end of the infirmary wing was a logical step. Over a year after writing the initial request and after innumerable visits, memos, demands, and negotiations, this step—which was clearly a responsibility of the Department of Correction to begin with—was carried out by a civilian welder, paid for by the research funds of the Prison Health Project. The gate, to this day, remains as a visible reminder to those who fought the battle of the labyrinthine ways of overlapping bureaucracies overseeing a constituency with no political clout.

At the end of his first year of work, Dr. Pastorello was voted Man of the Year by the prisoners of Walpole. He stayed two years, organizing an effective medical service by the sheer force of his integrity and determination. It was not long after he left that the system fell apart, leading to the later court action.

Less than a year after the project began, DellaPenna was successfully recruited by the New York City correctional system to become the first director of the revolutionary medical care system, operating under contract between the city of New York and Montefiore Hospital. After a few years, DellaPenna returned to civilian medicine in California having made important contributions in Massachusetts and New York. DellaPenna was part of the original group within the American Public Health Association that set the first prison health care standards. These were the basis for the standards now in effect throughout the nation for the accreditation of prisons.

WASHINGTON, D.C.

As if the administrative turmoil of Massachusetts were not bad enough, throughout the life of the Prison Health Project relations with Washington were strained. The federal Department of Health, Education, and Welfare was repeatedly reorganized during the early 1970s, and with each reorganization came a new project manager for the Prison Health Project and a new set of acronyms, filing regulations, budgetary constraints, and bureaucratic dilemmas. The Prison Health Project was conceived and established by the Office of Economic Opportunity, which had been set up during the early years of the Kennedy administration. In early 1972 when the contract was drawn up, President Nixon was running for reelection and rumors were widespread that the Nixon administration, on winning the election, would abandon the OEO. Such proved to be the case. The very month that the project began, its political support disappeared.

Among the many agencies that successively took over all or part of the oversight of the Prison Health Project were several administrators who were impressive in their knowledge and their dedication. Each of them had many other duties and none was exclusively dedicated to issues of prison health. Under the eagle eye of critical administration and legislative committees, at a time when social concerns were rapidly receding from the forefront of political activity, the original latitude, which was one of the strengths and weaknesses of the poverty program, was progressively constrained.

When the project was getting underway, administrative problems in Washington prevented funds from being released. The first federal payment did not arrive until 3 November 1972, three months after the project had been authorized to commence.

Federal control of the purse strings severely hampered operations. For example, an excellent psychiatrist who had worked at Charles Street Jail, setting up psychiatric screening, said that he would like to work on the Prison Health Project. At the time, his suggestion sounded like the answer to our prayers. The project sorely needed a psychiatrist and to have a psychiatrist with experience in the jails was more than we could hope for. Unfortunately, however, because of the strict interpretation of the contract written by Washington, the project could not find the money to pay him because he was not an office-based planner.

A year later, in October 1973, the Prison Health Project was dealt a crippling blow when the budget was cut from $306,000 to $225,000. Typically, the project was squeezed between the federal and state forces. The Massachusetts Executive Office of Human Services, using the bureaucratic argot of the day, said that the federal decision was "unacceptable." Of course, this rhetoric changed nothing. Despite all efforts to the contrary, the Prison Health Project was forced to run on a severely limited budget.

Accepting the reality of the budget cuts and the futility of depending on a confused federal mandate and a nearly bankrupt state, Prout tried to enlist private support for the project. Several large public foundations were at the time increasing their interest in broader health problems and the idea of restructuring the systems providing care to the public was becoming a major focus. The particular instance of providing better health care to prison inmates, however, was not attractive to them. Prout tried personal appeals to his friend John Knowles, president of the Rockefeller Foundation, but had no success. The Rockefeller, Carnegie, Ford, and Johnson Foundations all answered in effect that the Prison Health Project is a wonderful and timely venture but, unfortunately, not within the areas funded by their foundations.

CRISIS IN THE PROJECT

Every day brought crises. Coping with them was a matter of survival. Long-range planning, the supposed purpose of the project, was made impossible by the constant press of immediate problems. For example, before designing, testing, and implementing the model drug rehabilitation program, which was one of the main responsibilities of the project, and before reliable records and a plan of attack could be worked out, the project was faced with a drug crisis at Walpole State Prison. In 1973, of the 650 inmates at Walpole, almost 500 were being prescribed daily doses of Talwin, an addictive narcotic drug. It was being prescribed nominally for a variety of conditions. Original orders had been given by a series of physicians who came in to cover for short periods of time and under severe threat caved in and gave short-term prescriptions for Talwin. These would be renewed by the next physician who came in and was subjected to the same pressures from the inmates. To refuse writing the new prescription would involve the visiting physician at the least in a protracted and heated battle with the inmate and, at worst, to intimidation or even physical attack.

There being no medical records, indications for the original prescription were missing. The lack of privacy and security in the infirmary wing of the prison made it necessary to prepare for a large-scale riot if this medication was cut off "cold turkey." The likelihood of severe withdrawal symptoms on discontinuing Talwin abruptly had to be reckoned with.

On 12 April 1973, the supplies ran out and 500 Talwin-dependent prisoners were deprived of their supply. There was no alternative to prevent a probable riot than to get a supply of the drug into the prison immediately. Members of the project had inherited an impossible situation and, after consulting with state officials, decided to procure an emergency supply of the drug.

Two of the well-meaning people on the project and one of the state people involved in the drug program wanted to call a general meeting of the Walpole inmates so that they could talk to them reasonably about the dangers of addiction and then ask them to discontinue using the drug. This was a plan so naive as not to be seriously considered.

Things went from bad to worse. On 19 May, we received word that the pharmacy was about to be stormed and that a general riot would almost certainly follow. There was no overall prison emergency plan, nor was anyone on hand at Walpole to handle, even on an ad hoc basis, the growing emergency. Pastorello called Prout in the middle of the night, demanding that he come out to the prison. Why Prout? No one could find the commissioner of the Department of Correction or the director of the Office of Human Services that night.

Fortunately, the Prison Health Project had developed a detailed emergency plan to be put into effect in case of riot. Amazingly enough, the plan worked. At least the medical department was fully prepared when the riot began. In fact, the medical department appeared to be the only segment of the correctional system that was prepared to deal with the emergency.

The state police saved the situation by moving in promptly and efficiently to relieve the Walpole guards of any responsibility—or even right—to restore order. The state police actually kept the correctional officers away from the scene until they regained control.

Both of the physicians threatened to quit over the lack of administrative firmness and general lack of support. Prout feared that he was about to become, for lack of anyone else to do the job, medical director for both Walpole and Norfolk. In the electrifying atmosphere of impending riot, there were many conflicting statements and plans. One involved giving Prout one of the state automobiles equipped with a radio so that he could be kept informed at all times of developments in the crisis. When he got into his newly issued automobile, he found much to his relief that the radio did not work at all.

TROUBLES

In the meantime, the Department of Public Health had committed the project to delivering medical care within the prisons. The Department of Correction controlled such budget as existed for prison medicine, however, so that the Prison Health Project had no way of funding the efforts even if the project could agree on a clear course of action.

By the summer of 1973, it was clear to all those who felt that they had a stake in the operation of the Prison Health Project—Prout, Bicknell, Goldmark, the federal Department of Health, Education, and Welfare, and the Department of Correction—that an authoritarian, systems-oriented administrator with experience in dealing with the federal government was an absolute necessity.

For more than a year, the project had gone off in many directions, inefficiently spending time, energy, and money on ventures that had to be left half-finished because of wrangles with Washington over their propriety and because of confusion of goals within the project itself. Education, training, and placement became key efforts of the Prison Health Project. In the eyes of the commonwealth, however, staffing of medical facilities in the prisons, security, drug abuse, and many other insoluble problems all were referred to the Prison Health Project. As so often was the case, it was not clear under whose department this effort was going to become a reality.

Without a strong administrator, the Prison Health Project would continue to stagger under the weight of problems confronting it. Prout himself was frustrated by his own efforts to please so many masters. His sense of failure was deepened when the OEO staffers in Washington said that unless the project quickly found an administrator, the entire program would be terminated.

Increasingly, Prout came to realize that the high ideals and political naivete of the staff often interfered with their practical usefulness. OEO was defunct by this time. Times had changed. If the project staff continued without taking into account these social and political changes, they would be the instruments of their own undoing. If the Prison Health Project were to survive, it would need to change with the political tone of the Nixon administration. At the very least, the project would need to put its house in order.

After interviewing several candidates who were found to be unacceptable to the contract supervisor, Prout appointed Frank Chasen to the job. This was Prout's decision and, unlike weighty decisions in the past, was not submitted to a vote of the project staff. Chasen was appointed by fiat.

Chasen was a well-organized administrator whose manner was guaranteed to offend members of the project staff. He was an academic with a business background. He understood economics, law, and management. He prided himself on his nonemotional approach to problems and saw little good in doctrinaire or polemical approaches. Chasen proclaimed that he had been hired to keep the Prison Health Project running smoothly, not to root out injustice. He felt that his job was to keep the project on the narrow path defined in its contract with HEW. Any of the staff who would try to suspend or broadly interpret the mandates of the grant to the Prison Health Project ran directly into Chasen's stolid opposition.

Chasen's reports pleased the administrators at the Massachusetts Health Research Institute and the project officer at HEW. His appointment, however, changed the tone of the Prison Health Project. Before his coming, staff meeting were enthusiastic, boisterous free-for-alls. After his arrival, meetings became tense and even hostile. This was not directly Chasen's doing, but rather his presence brought to the surface irreconcilable differences in style and intent lay just beneath the surface from the outset of the project.

The battle lines were now drawn. In a 16 January 1974 memorandum regarding the future of the Prison Health Project to Prout from Clapp, Cyrus, Dettmann, Mantone, Robinson, and Torrey of the project staff, the group focused on Chasen as the source of "the deterioration of staff morale and effectiveness." They blamed "his adverse effect on the goals and operation" of the project and threatened that their "continuation as a staff without the removal of F. Chasen is now in question."

In this memo, the staff raised "several questions . . . of more immediate importance" regarding the future of the entire project. In particular, the dissident staff asked the following questions:

Are we backing away from our original mandate via the Madoff Report to form an autonomous Office of Special Health Services accountable to medical people, the larger community, and prisoners?

Are we backing away from the necessary and hard work to create an Office of Health Services . . . that provides more in the realm of health than the physician sick line?

Why have we failed thus far in our second year to get a redefinition, reaffirmation of project goals, priorities, and actions, through a process of collaborative decision making? Has our office policy been unilaterally changed to a top-down decision-making management— with communication, cooperation, and consultation among the total staff no longer welcomed or accepted?

The group conceded that, except for the "non-negotiable demand" that Frank Chasen be removed from his position, "mutual dialogue, trust, and accountability" will resolve "the present impasse." "In any event," they concluded, "February 15, 1974 stands as the outside limit of our capacity to endure the continuation of the status quo." The memo from the staff was widely disseminated, including sending copies to members of the inmates' councils.

The next day, Prout replied with his own memo to the staff's "self-serving and potentially dangerous" move. Prout interpreted their action as an attempt "to stir up inmates against some people who have been trying (perhaps, I admit, not very successfully) to help them."

The crisis had come. In their memo to Prout, the staff maintained that "mutual dialogue" would resolve the present impasse. Prout, however, disagreed, as he wrote in his own memo, "that more talk will solve all these problems. None of you are naive enough to believe this. Certainly I don't." Consequently, to quell the growing discontent and to put an immediate end to the rebellion of the staff, Prout asked Sunny Robinson to leave the project. "Others may resign if they wish," Prout wrote.

Prout continued his defense: "The failure of this project, after 16 months and thousands of dollars, to produce specific accomplishments in this line has produced great criticism. Frank's and my efforts to channel the appropriate persons' work in these lines have met with great resistance. I find that problems of public statements, personnel policy, research, even the dates of office meetings, hours of working, have been taken over by various members of the Project independently. Democracy is one thing—chaos is another."

With that rebuttal, Prout wrote to the governor and the commissioners, offering to resign. His letter explained:

Most of you know that I have been under great pressure from many directions, apparently irreconcilable, from the inmates for more services, more doctors, more medics, more medications—things which despite our best efforts, have not been forthcoming because of the lack of state money. I have also been under great pressure from them to take federal grant money and apply it to direct services in the institutions. . . . On another side, pressure has come from Washington to produce tangible research and evaluation reports and a plan to be replicated in other areas. [Meanwhile, from the Office of Human Services have come] demands for complete physical examination screening in Walpole when we have not the money or circumstances to retain medics or to keep up with the daily sick call.

The Department of Correction had asked the project to deliver more services, to find competent physicians, and not to send inmates to outside hospitals. "From the thrust of the Madoff Report and from my own conscience as a physician, I must continue to send certain persons to outside hospitals for medical care," Prout wrote.

Pressure had been most intense from the staff of the project. Prout acknowledged that Frank Chasen has been "direct and at times forceful and even abrasive" in his dealings with the staff so that "many people feel threatened and angered." But the most dangerous aspect of the conflict, in Prout's view, was that the staff sent their memo to the Inmates Medical Advisory Committee, "which I can only regard as a somewhat demogogic action and one which is going to make it awfully difficult in the future."

The public members of the inmates advisory committees in general sided with the dissidents. One of them, Bonnie Gorman, R.N., wrote to Prout on 19 January 1974, in an open letter, that "the crisis is at hand. The original goals and objectives [of the Prison Health Project] seem somehow to have been adjusted to those of the commonwealth—NO CHANGE, BUSINESS AS USUAL," she wrote. Gorman especially objected to the "obvious retaliatory measures" taken against Sunny Robinson. "I implore you—CHOOSE LIFE, CHOOSE PROGRESS."

On 21 January 1974, six staff members resigned. "The same disagreements about philosophy and project accountability which have caused [Sunny Robinson's] departure have made it necessary for each of us to terminate our employment at the Prison Health Project concurrently with Sunny's termination date." Richard W. Clapp, Catherine Cyrus, Sonia H. Dettmann, William A. Mantone, Bernadette McClain, and Evelyn J. Torrey resigned.

Ten days later, on 1 February 1974, the dissident staff released a statement to the press at five o'clock on a Friday afternoon. It read as follows:

Today, one half of the Prison Health staff is resigning because the Project has failed to meet its mandate to correct health abuses in prisons. In 1971, a state investigation of prison health services documented that Massachusetts had failed to provide decent health care for prisoners. The Prison Health Project was subsequently formed to take immediate steps to: (1) insure that every prisoner would receive adequate, complete medical care; (2) correct problems of poor sanitation, housing, and food, and end isolation and segregation of prisoners; (3) create a coordinated prison health care system independent of the Department of Correction.

We charge that the Project has failed to move beyond a bandaid approach to prison medical care. While the prisoners cry out about isolation, segregation, food, sanitation, and beatings, the Project has failed to publicly protect or prevent such abuses.

- Instead of playing a watch-dog role on drug research in the state prisons, the Project administration has facilitated researchers and left the prisons dependent on them for part of needed medical services. This would not be done by serious health advocates.
- While serious questions exist about the proposed New England Regional prison, in relation to violation of confidentiality of medical records and mind-altering drugs and techniques, the Project has taken no initiative to prevent those abuses. This is not the position of genuine health advocates.
- Instead of taking a position against sending women to MCI Bridgewater, where it is widely accepted that no one gets good care, project administrators have vacillated and may allow this to happen. This is not the position of serious health advocates.
- Project administration has not adequately supported the staff's efforts to develop health training and work-release programs. This is not the position of people seriously interested in using health resources to aid re-integration.
- While there is a system-wide health advisory committee, and institutional health committees made up of prisoners and community people, the Project administration has excluded them from policy-making decisions.

The news release from the dissidents continued: "A Prison Health Project which fails to address these grave health issues is not meeting its responsibilities to prisoners or the larger community. The absence of such a clear position of health-related problems has left the Project subject to the regressive directions of the Department of Correction, contrary to the Project's charge to be an independent health service. The efforts of half the staff to move the Project to some of these larger concerns have been repeatedly stymied by Project administration. We therefore find it necessary to resign and move outside the Project to function as its critics."

Prout replied to the statements of the dissident staff in a written statement of his own on 4 February 1974. "Some of the statements are untruths, or half-truths," he wrote, "and others blame the Project for not doing things which it was not supposed to do. The justifiable anger at the shortcomings of the system and its abuses was turned on the Project rather than the system."

Then in his point-by-point rebuttal Prout responded to the criticisms ventilated by the dissidents. The acrimonious exchange between Prout and the dissident staff is instructive, for in it the two sides express in writing the heart of the conflict that tore the project apart and that typifies the emotional responses of the American people to prisons and prisoners.

According to the dissidents, the charge to the Prison Health Project was "to insure that every prisoner would receive adequate, complete medical care, to correct problems of poor sanitation, housing and food, and [to] end isolation and segregation." This, Prout pointed out, was not the case. The terms of the OEO grant stipulated that the Prison Health Project was for research and development of a model health care system for prisoners in Massachusetts under the Department of Public Health. The project was to study a plan for handling drug abuse problems in the prison system. One part of this drug abuse program was to be a model prerelease program at Shirley. Finally, the charge to the project was to train and place inmates in health careers.

The project mandate did not include ending segregation, insuring adequate health care, or correcting problems of sanitation, housing, and food. It is a clear failure of these well-meaning individuals that they could not separate medical activities, in which they were expert and invited to participate by the OEO grant, from correctional activities.

The reference to a regional prison was made up of whole cloth from scraps of information coming from a New England governor's conference. It had to do with the empty prison in the U.S. government's Portsmouth Naval Hospital, located in Kittery, Maine. The suggestion had been made that the overcrowding in all New England state prisons could be relieved by using this very large facility. Nothing ever came of these discussions, and as of 1988, the prison was still unused. Nowhere had any discussion taken place having the slightest connection with confidentiality or the role of the Department of Correction or the Prison Health Project in promoting this idea.

The accusation that the Prison Health Project had abandoned the goal of moving medical services away from Correction was unfounded. At that time, it remained the intent of the project to establish a separate Division of Special Health Services (Prison Medicine) under a full-time physician, with a director who would report to both the Department of Correction and the Department of Public Health.

The charge that the project had taken a "bandaid approach" reflected the intention of the dissident staff to make sweeping changes.

On the subject of research being carried out on prisoners, the facts were that only one research project was under way, at Norfolk Prison. This research was carried out with the advice and consent of all approving authorities, including the Inmate Medical Advisory Committees. The firm conducting this research was reliable and had been conducting similar research for many years. The inmate volunteers were paid for their participation in the studies and the firm also paid for the services of a much-needed consulting physician one day a week at Norfolk Hospital. "The question of whether or not research of any description should be done on inmates is still a matter of debate," wrote Prout. "If there were a system where the medical care was all that it should be and the prisoners had enough funds for the simple necessities of life, I myself would probably oppose research in prisons."

On the subject of women being sent to Bridgewater, many meetings of the project had been devoted to the question of what to do with violent women. Four to six women a year were committed to Framingham with such violent behavior that they could not be kept in that institution. In the past, such people were sent to one of the state mental hospitals, but under the new commitment laws, these hospitals declined to take such patients. The question then became whether to staff a special unit at Framingham, which would be empty most of the time, or to send these few violent women somewhere else. If somewhere else, Bridgewater was the only alternative.

Actually only one woman was sent to Bridgewater, by an angry judge who defied the law. Prout himself visited Bridgewater and interviewed the woman who had been sent there. She seemed to be doing unusually well.

LEGACIES OF THE PRISON HEALTH PROJECT

Prout said in his letter responding to the dissidents, "Part of the anger and bitterness has arisen because this was a research and development project and because of its nature, it was never promised by the government, the authorities or me that we could remedy all the deficiencies of the correctional system or supply operating money for a good medical department."

The Prison Health Project went riding off in three directions at the same time, following very different mandates. (1) From the people in the Department of Public Health came the order to throw out the "incompetent and uncaring" people in the Department of Correction and to put prison health under the direction of the Department of Public Health. However, when the Prison Health Project put the issue to them during the two years of the project, the Department of Public Health protested in many ways that they could not possibly take responsibility for prison health. (2) A second mandate was to train the prisoners in health professions to serve as medics and technicians while in prison, preparing for employment in the health professions upon release from prison. Experience, as we shall see, proved this plan to be wholly unworkable. (3) A third was to set up a model drug rehabilitation program. There was no money or legal authority to carry this out, no agreement then as to how to rehabilitate drug addicts.

One of the recommendations of the Madoff Report was not incorporated in the grant to the Prison Health Project: to consider health problems of the guards. This was a noble but insufficiently considered idea. It was neither requested nor accepted by the guards. Experiences elsewhere have since confirmed that the medical care of the correctional staff should be kept separate from that of the prisoners.

Under Prout were young, idealistic, angry people who felt that the system was evil and unregenerate. To some of them, the project was seen as an entering wedge whereby they could fight the authorities, befriend the prisoners, and possibly even get some people released from prison. These people worked long, hard, and earnestly. Gradually, however, it was obvious that there were limits to the objectives. The Prison Health Project could not satisfy everyone's personal and political needs. Nor could it satisfy the conflicting desires of society and inmates.

On 31 December 1974, the project disbanded. The only tangible and permanent progress made by the project came in the final few months, with a truncated but unified staff. Working then with Dr. Donald Scherl in the Office of Human Services, the Office of Correctional Health Services in the Department of Correction was established; it has worked satisfactorily ever since. The other important legacies were to legitimize and standardize the role of medics, establish standards, and most important, demonstrate what can and cannot be accomplished in a prison health care setting. It became obvious that even a rare, strong individual physician, such as Pastorello and DellaPenna, can only partially succeed in running an acceptable health care service without strong structural support, a disciplined prison, and constant vigilance. The improvements brought about by Pastorello, DellaPenna, and the project promptly dissolved when they departed.

3
The Judicial Approach

The Prison Health Project was unfortunately a quixotic effort because the small group of hard-working, highly motivated and bright liberal activists set out on their mission without first garnering the requisite legislative, financial, and judicial backing. Their motives became confused when their good intentions collided with the political and social realities of prison reform. They turned their frustration and anger inward and, in the process, destroyed the chief asset of the Prison Health Project—the clarity of their reformer's zeal and the sense of joint participation in a good cause. With that went all hope of changing the system, for the obverse of zeal is despair.

In 1977, three years after the Prison Health Project dissolved in disarray, another group in Massachusetts launched an entirely new effort to reform prison health care, urged on by different motives and employing far different tactics. This time, the results were significantly different. Following the lead in other jurisdictions, an aggressive lawyer approached the matter of improving prison health care by the judicial route and this approach seems to have produced a much more profound and lasting change than strictly medical efforts guided by physicians or (worse) do-good efforts driven by undisciplined sentiment. As the judicial approach seems, at this time, to be the most effective one, it is worth examining the painful steps by which its successes have been achieved.

It is hard to separate cause from effect here. The standards developed by the AMA and other professional organizations (see

87

chapter 7) vastly improved the legal means of redressing wrongs in the prison health system by providing an understandable framework within which to work toward achievable goals. By the same token, the stronger civil rights laws and regulations under which court cases could be developed strengthened the need for cogent, comprehensive, and credible standards of adequate health care. No matter whose contribution to advances in prison health care might be the greater, the fact is that the confluence of medical and legal developments through the 1970s and up to the present has significantly changed attitudes concerning prison health care. Changed attitudes have also altered the strategies for reforming prison medicine.

As the 1970s gave way to the 1980s, Massachusetts in particular, and the country at large, underwent deep political and philosophical changes. This was a period of reaction to the welfare-oriented social planning of the 1960s and early 1970s. Richard Nixon was reelected, the Congress moved firmly to the right, and in Massachusetts two liberal governors—one a Republican and one a Democrat—were replaced by a hard-line, ultraconservative Democrat. "Safety nets," as they were to be called in a later administration, were being pulled out from under all but the most self-reliant and self-possessed segments of society. Sympathy for prisoners was waning.

This waning of sentiment is not itself a bad thing; for, as we have pointed out, although sentiments change from one era to another, they seem at the time to be completely right and unassailable to those under their sway. Thus in relatively recent theories of prison reform, religious sentiment has given way to psychological, sociological, environmental, and now medical models. These models rose and fell with changing intellectual and political fashions, their successes and failures having little to do with their practicality or truth. Each model provided a partial theory of criminal behavior. Each had a modicum of reasonableness; none held the whole truth. Each model did, in its time, provide a rationale for programs to define and deal with criminal behavior.

Physicians, clergymen, professors, politicians, and social activists have tried for years, in various ways, to improve health care of prisoners, but the few changes they effect have proved to be ad hoc and too often transient. The dramatic and systematic improvements of the last decade have generally not been the result of new programs instituted by such public-spirited groups as the Prison Health Project or by national organizations like the American Medical Association or the American Bar Association. Nor have they been a direct result of federal, state, or local executive or legislative action. Where idealistic physicians and public-spirited reformers have failed utterly, pragmatic lawyers and jurists have had at least partial success.

Depending on the law is different from depending on theology, sociology, or medicine because, unlike these other intellectual disciplines, the law emphasizes procedure. Science and theology have their sacred rituals, to be sure, but the orderly processes of science or theology are designed to bring human beings to greater knowledge of something else. Law, on the other hand, is dedicated to perfecting the process itself. Other social goods may devolve from defining and exercising *due process*, but improving the procedure and enjoying the good are not the same thing.

Thus it was that, in shifting tactics, reform through the judicial process brought the greatest promise of a happy outcome. Good will and good intentions were far less relevant to the case than the clear question of how the case was to be prosecuted, what legal precedents could be found, and what basic principles of law could be marshaled to make the case. As a result, the rhetoric of reform was changed dramatically.

Aggrieved parties in America have always had recourse to the courts, but prisoners have been at a disadvantage in enjoying this legal recourse. Lacking education, subscribing to the values of a social underclass, and often suffering from mental and emotional disorders as well, prison inmates have found themselves confronted by severely limited choices. In addition to these socioeconomic factors, there is the additional fact that because prisoners have been deprived of many civil rights by virtue of their incarceration, the status of their remaining rights is often unclear. Finally, in a purely practical sense, prison inmates often lack the money required to carry their grievances to court.

A major advance in strengthening the civil rights of prison inmates came in 1976, when the United States Congress amended the civil rights laws to provide that successful plaintiffs in a civil rights case could have their legal fees paid by the losing party. If necessary, the plaintiff's lawyers could even come into court to ask the judge to issue an order forcing the losing party to pay any reasonable fees incurred in preparing and presenting the case. Before the civil rights law was extended in this way, the substantial legal costs of bringing a complaint to court inhibited plaintiffs and attorneys from entering civil rights cases. With the possibility of recovering substantial legal fees and damages, lawyers and plaintiffs took up civil rights cases with renewed vigor. The chief impetus for such legislation was the struggle for black civil rights, but as a result, other disenfranchised groups, including prison inmates, enjoyed the benefit of the law.

This simple ruling has changed the course of prison medicine as no liberal, well-intentioned, sentimental reform movement could. Although there were larger profits to be made in other areas of the law, the possibility of getting paid at all for time and services rendered in defense of prisoners' rights allowed at least some of the major law firms in the country to take on prison cases. For the first time, *pro bono* work was not strictly charity. This was also a sign of how vigorously some federal lawmakers intended to strengthen civil rights legislation.[1]

BEGINNINGS OF THE WALPOLE CASE

To spread the risk among the law firms, several of the most socially minded law firms in Boston formed a clearing committee to refer appropriate civil rights cases to the participating firms. It was through this committee that the Walpole case originally came to the Boston firm of Palmer and Dodge and to Scott Lewis. In 1976, Palmer and Dodge had been appointed to represent an inmate who was challenging the fact that he was at the universally hated Massachusetts Correctional Institution at Walpole.[2] This inmate would have preferred to spend his time at the more tolerable Norfolk. For Scott Lewis, the Walpole inmate's case was a good opportunity to work for his ideals while developing his skills as a courtroom advocate and gaining visibility within the legal community. "But in the course of just coming to know this gentleman," said Scott Lewis, "I learned of some extraordinarily bad medical care that he had gotten and some badly needed care that he had not gotten."[3]

Another of Boston's most-respected law firms had already begun work on a class action case at Walpole. But, as a representative of the firm told Lewis, that firm was obligated to drop the case since it had acted as special attorneys general for the Department of Public Health, a potential defendant in the Walpole case, and thus would have a conflict of interest. The case was offered to Lewis. The seniors at Palmer and Dodge gave their approval, and Lewis jumped at the opportunity. "We really didn't talk about prison medical care in the administration of that law firm," he said. "But it was an interesting example of how a law firm can meet the needs and desires of a junior person. I was a third-year litigation associate at the time. I was given authority to prosecute the case and to be in charge of running it."

The early stages of the case were developed by Arlene Marcus, who served with Lewis as co-counsel. She was a staff lawyer at the nonprofit reform organization known as the Prisoners' Rights Project when the case was begun. (The Prisoners' Rights Project is now the Massachusetts Correctional Legal Services.) Walpole was originally her case. For the first three years, Arlene Marcus played a major role in directing and shaping it. She collected the plaintiffs, decided on the underlying issues, and teased out the legal implications. According to Scott Lewis, "She deserves the credit for having thought it out. It is her brainchild." Arlene Marcus was to continue to assist in shaping and directing the conduct of the case; but as time went on, her role in the case gradually diminished.

Scott Lewis and Arlene Marcus started the suit in 1977, devoting many months to the pretrial discovery phase of the case. *Discovery* is the legal process of finding out just what happened. It is a more or less orderly procedure of collecting documents and depositions. Discovery in the Walpole case was extremely difficult, as it turned out, because the Department of Correction had few medical records and what records they did have were poorly organized. Lewis and Marcus went to the Department of Correction and to the medical department at Walpole, reviewing their files and taking depositions from Dr. Edmund Nevs and Mark Gallant, a medical assistant.

Their first and primary target was the Department of Correction, the agency that had the most obvious legal and common-sense obligation to provide adequate medical care at Walpole. On looking into the case further, however, Lewis and Marcus decided to bring two other agencies into the case as defendants— the Department of Mental Health and the Department of Public Health.

The Department of Mental Health was brought in, not because the case was challenging the delivery of mental health services to the general prison population, but because a statute peculiar to Massachusetts says that the medical and psychiatric health of inmates who are kept in segregated units must be monitored regularly by the Department of Mental Health. Lewis and Marcus felt that this surveillance, mandated by statute, was not being done at MCI, Walpole.

Similarly, a 1911 statute charged the Department of Public Health with the responsibility of drafting prison health regulations setting forth details of the entrance physical examinations. The Department of Public Health had not carried out its obligation almost seventy years later. When the Prison Health Project developed its own health assessment forms in 1973, setting standards for the initial physical examination, personnel at MCI, Walpole, did not follow their protocol either. "That was a case we could not lose," said Scott Lewis. "Whatever happened, that case was open and shut from the very beginning."

"The Department was not happy with what we were doing and they felt that our suit was absolutely without merit. That was their public position." The Department of Correction resented the public scrutiny of its activities. They maintained that the suit was without merit because whatever deficiencies might have existed at one time in the prison medical system administered by the Department of Correction no longer existed. They were arguing, in effect, that the medical system has been fine and, in any event, its problems had been solved.

An internal analysis of the situation had led the Department of Correction to conclude that their own physicians, state medical employees serving at Massachusetts state prisons, simply were not good enough. In light of this internal study, the Department of Correction did begin thinking about improving the prison medical system, but, as Lewis, Marcus, and other observers of the Massachusetts prison system realized, without constant scrutiny from the outside, there was little likelihood of any lasting changes being made.

THE WALPOLE PROBLEM

The Massachusetts Correctional Institution at Walpole (MCI, Walpole) was conceived in haste and has remained a source of trouble ever since. As we have mentioned, the architect's plans for Walpole were used because they already existed and not because they were appropriate for the site or for the purpose of the prison.

Walpole was built to replace the old Charlestown State Prison. State Senator Lewis Parkhurst (Sixth Middlesex District) wrote, in a pamphlet dated 1933,

> That the Charlestown State Prison has long been considered a disgrace to our State is a matter of record which I wish once more to call to the attention of the Governor and members of the Legislature. In 1880, when the Concord Reformatory was built, the Prison was deemed unfit for futher use and remained vacant for six years, being used for storage purposes only. In 1920, Sanford Bates, Commissioner of Correction . . . said in his annual report, "The present structure was built in 1805. It is antiquated, out of date, and hard to keep clean. It is in a congested and dirty location. There are no adequate hospital facilities. There is no congregate dining-room, with the result that men are obliged to eat all their meals in their cells. This is unhygienic, wasteful of food, and conducive to unclean conditions. The absence from the cells of any kind of plumbing makes necessary the obnoxious and unhealthy "bucket system," and in general the cell block construction is not conducive to health. (Quoted in Parkhurst, 1939, p. 25)

Perhaps the strongest argument for destroying the Charlestown Prison was economic. In the words of Senator Parkhurst,

Strict economy in national, state, and municipal governments is now demanded by the people of the country. The extravagant and often-times unnecessary expenses must be curtailed, so that the great burden of taxation now borne by every one in the land may be reduced. Can the State of Massachusetts longer afford to use nearly ten acres of land in Charlestown—in the midst of the business and transportation section of the city, valued at one dollar per square foot by the assessors of Boston—when it owns about a thousand acres of land in Norfolk, worth, unimproved, not more than $15.00 an acre?

The economic argument had been around for quite a long time. In 1921, Edwin S. Webster, Commissioner on State Administration and Expenditure, argued for abandoning the state prison at Charlestown because it was "obsolete." The clincher to his argument, however, was, "The property on which the prison is located has a value for other purposes which has been estimated between $750,000 and $1,000,000."

Moral and economic arguments fell on deaf ears until prison riots forced the issue. There had been terrible riots at Charlestown—so serious in fact, that the National Guard was called out, and they came fully armed and supported by tanks. The inmates made a desperate stand in what turned out to be a bloody confrontation.

"An envelope manufacturer got appointed Commissioner of Corrections," recalled Howard Gill.

He had heard about the destruction of Charlestown and ran down to Washington to ask if they didn't have a plan. An architect from the Federal Bureau had been playing for some time with a plan for a maximum-security prison. It was just a plaything with him. This envelope manufacturer came in and asked for a plan for an institution and they handed him this. He accepted it and came back to Massachusetts to tell the Legislature that the Federal Bureau had recommended this plan. Massachusetts accepted it on his say so; and that was the beginning of Walpole. It was a monstrosity. It's a terrible place.

During the turmoil of the early 1970s, Walpole Prison was frequently the scene of violence and the subject of journalistic scrutiny. Miguel Trinidad, vice president of the Walpole Inmates'

Organization (member of the National Prison Reform Association), organized a demonstration of about one hundred Walpole
inmates, who marched peaceably carrying placards proclaiming,
"In Sympathy with Prisoners in Rhode Island and New Hamp-
shire," "Support Prison Reform," and "Give Prison Reform a
Chance" (*Boston Globe*, 9 June 1973). Jeremy Taylor wrote in the
Globe (16 April 1973) that "idleness is visible everywhere" at
Walpole. The story carried the headline, "Walpole: The prison
where there's nothing to do."

Inmates did find something to do: in the period between 1
September and 2 December 1973, there were three fatal stab-
bings at Walpole. On Friday night, 19 May 1973, 551 inmates at
Walpole rioted for twelve hours, storming through corridors and
cell blocks. Before a force of 180 heavily armed state police could
quell the riot, the rampaging inmates did more than $800,000 of
damage to the prison. (Prout's role in controlling the riot is described in the previous chapter.) Ray Richard and Stephen
Wermiel reported for the *Globe* (20 April 1973) that "the tension
at the prison is heightened by the daily exchange of charges that
inmates are running the prison, that drugs and weapons are
spread throughout the building, that prostitution and homosexual
rape abound, and that inmates are bribing employees."

In February 1974, Judge W. Arthur Garrity ordered Magistrate
Peter W. Princi to hear a suit by Gene Tremblay, an inmate at
Walpole, charging that he was held in segregation in the infamous
Walpole Cell Block 10 for six months, from 5 August 1973 to 14
February 1974, without knowing the reason why. Superintendent
Douglas H. Vinzant and Frank Howard, director of departmental
segregation, said that Tremblay was confined to Cell Block 10
because his life was in danger.

As an editorial in the *Globe* asserted, "the time is long overdue
to establish a permanent impartial body to look into prison problems and disputes" (22 April 1974). Gary McMillan wrote in the
Globe (11 August 1974), "The inmates, whose disgust at unkept
promises led to the riot, have adopted an attitude of seething
watchfulness." They had seen many changes of personnel and
philosophy. In December 1972, Superintendent Raymond Porell
began a five-week shakedown and lockup at Walpole, at the very

time the then commissioner John O. Boone was trying to institute liberal reforms. Porell resigned. Another Department of Correction regular, Waikevitch, took his job and shortly after announced his own general lockup. The result: the riot of May 1973 and a year of confusion. Then, on 21 June 1974, Boone himself was fired.

Joseph Rosenbloom wrote in his *Globe* column the next day "Political Circuit," "Boone had a folksy, sometimes inscrutable manner about him. As commissioner, he was long on guts, short on tact. . . . Since Boone's departure, the wheels of reform at Walpole have come to a grinding halt. . . . The inmates sit in the cells day after day, bitter and idle." (*Boston Globe*, 12 August 1974).

Problems were legion. The new commissioner, Frank Hall, decried the conditions at Walpole. "It's a badly designed institution, outmoded," he was quoted as saying (*Boston Globe*, 15 June 1974). "We don't have the kind of money or staff to provide programs that would have an impact." Recalling the May riot, Hall said, "If that was a maximum-security prison, why did its inner control room crumble? Why could men knock through the walls? If that [construction] was done right the first time, the state wouldn't have to come in and spend a million dollars. That's what we're stuck with."

Another editorial in the *Globe* (14 December 1974) described "the Walpole problem." "The Walpole problem," according to the editorial, "is as old as the intitution, a monstrosity which never should have been built. In it men are jammed together in a harsh environment which seems to have been designed to irritate them. Most are given little or nothing to do and have only their eventual freedom to look forward to." In conclusion, the editorial says, "the most rational" solution to the Walpole problem would be "to close it down tomorrow."

Three full years later (19 October 1977), State Senators William Owens (D–Mattapan), Jack Backman (D–Brookline), and Doris Bunte (D–Roxbury) visited Walpole. "We found rats in the cells . . . debris all over the floors . . . things so hazardous that there is a chance of a hepatitis outbreak," said Owens. Bunte deplored the "health hazardous conditions" as well.

Discounting the political rhetoric of the visitors and the political bias of the *Globe*, the fact remains that Walpole was an ongoing problem throughout the 1970s. Conditions at the prison were deplorable by any measure of decency; the public agencies responsible for remedying the bad situation at the prison were not up to the task. Then, too, these were special times. Civil rights agitation had extended into the prisons so that prison inmates were no longer willing to endure the privations and deprivations that former generations of inmates might have tolerated in sullen silence. This was a vocal generation of inmates, ready to exercise their civil rights and even eager for the fight.

PREPARATION FOR THE WALPOLE CASE

During its all-too-brief existence, the Prison Health Project had surveyed the medical situation at Walpole, along with other Massachusetts prisons in 1972 and 1973. As a result of this survey, the Prison Health Project made what nearly everyone acknowledges were significant improvements in the quality of medical care at Walpole and, to some degree, in the structure of medical services throughout the Massachusetts prison system. The greatest contribution the Prison Health Project made to improving health care at Walpole had been to recruit and support the heroic Doctor Ernest Pastorello, who was there from 1973 to 1975. But after he left and the Prison Health Project was disbanded in 1974, despite the best efforts of outside organizations to lobby for setting up systems to monitor health care at the prison, the medical care system at Walpole quickly collapsed as well. The place, according to Scott Lewis, "was an unmitigated disaster." There was strong evidence that prison inmates were running the Medical Service Department.

By 1977, the medical department was a shambles. The physician at Walpole, attacked on professional and administrative grounds, was in poor health and died during the course of the litigation. In the summer of 1977, the Prisoners' Rights Project recognized that there was a pattern of serious complaints at Walpole. Inmates complained that they could not gain access to medical treatment at Walpole and that the quality of treatment they did eventually receive was woefully inadequate. Arlene Marcus and her assistants surveyed the inmates, getting about six hundred responses. They also carefully reviewed the medical situations of dozens of inmates. On the basis of this survey, the Prisoners' Rights Project concluded that there was a systemic failure at Walpole Prison.

"Systemic failure" was a daring new legal argument to introduce to the Walpole case. Marcus, Lewis, and the Prisoners' Rights Project were arguing that the system was at fault at Walpole and not merely the individuals. In 1976, the United States Supreme Court had ruled that "deliberate indifference" to the serious medical needs of an inmate established a violation of the U.S. Constitution. Court opinions after that, principally in the Second Circuit, indicated that the constitutional test applied to an individual inmate who just got ignored by the system as well as to inmates who were treated with malice or systematic neglect. Consequently, in the fall of 1977, Lewis and Marcus decided to base their case on what they came to call "systematic evidence." These two lawyers knew that individual evidence, presented case by case, of inmates not getting the medical attention they deserved would obscure the hard, clear issues in the unending tangle of details. Systematic evidence, in contrast, would go directly to the heart of the issue.

The strategy of developing systematic evidence was effective for another reason, too—it elevated the case to the level of constitutional principle, legal obligation, and medical attention. Any of the individual inmates involved in the case might be a pathological liar, openly set upon making a mockery of the Department of Correction, or simply trying to get a day in court away from terrors and tedium of Walpole. The lawyers developing the Walpole case had to recognize the fact that they were dealing with unreliable characters whose motivation often was far from selfless. Marcus and Lewis deftly sidestepped these problems of developing the case by making it a cornerstone of their development that the case was larger and more significant than any of the single sad stories one might hear in taking depositions.

"We weren't about to commit resources of that scale to try to help eight people," said Lewis. "We thought we could aid everybody if we structured the case, factually and legally, on a systematic basis rather than on an ad hoc basis." The vagaries of individual medical circumstances really had nothing to do at all with the case. It was largely irrelevant whether any particular plaintiff had any particular problem. He just had to have enough of a problem to gain admission to the court case. "We did not want to talk about whether Mr. X's stomach cancer had been misdiagnosed. We wanted to talk about how does somebody get help when he says he is in pain."

That was a fundamental decision and a significant departure from tradition.

THE LEGAL TEAM

The legal staff preparing the Walpole case had the benefit of many people's help. Four consultants were especially important. Most studies of prison health have been based on departmental reports, reviews of medical records, and secondary sources. The studies in preparation for the Walpole case, in contrast, were based on firsthand, direct investigation by physicians from Harvard Medical School, Dieter Koch-Weser, George Lamb, and the medical students working with them, as well as occasional expert consultation from Dr. Curtis Prout and Dr. Barbara Starrett.

Dieter Koch-Weser, then chairman of the Harvard Medical School Department of Social and Preventive Medicine, and George Lamb (called Sandy by his colleagues), a pediatrician trained in public health, agreed to do what would surely be the hardest work of the project. Koch-Weser and Lamb spent an entire summer at Walpole with some Harvard medical students as helpers, studying the quality of medical care at Walpole in the greatest detail. They reviewed fifty randomly selected medical records and another twenty or thirty medical records selected by the lawyers. Koch-Weser and Lamb also examined inmates, reviewed their medical histories, and did everything but actually treat them.

The fourth consultant was Dr. Barbara Starrett, then in medical practice in New York and recognized as one of the leading experts on prison medical care. She was running the Rikers Island (New York) medical department for the New York Department of Correction on a contract originally designed by Dr. Richard DellaPenna, formerly of the Massachusetts system.

Scott Lewis and the legal staff had finished collecting the facts in the spring of 1979. They then decided upon their legal strategy, bringing an important issue before the court. Lewis and Marcus had asked the court not only to order the Department of Correction to make changes in medical service at Walpole but also to put to a jury the question of awarding money to the inmates who had been deprived of medical care in violation of their constitutional rights. Their legal theory was that each inmate in the case should be given a per diem payment in compensation for being deprived of his constitutional right per se. In this assertion, Lewis and Marcus relied on case law and academic legal writing.

Precedent existed for paying the aggrieved inmates a per diem for deprivation of their constitutional rights. The anti–Viet Nam War demonstrators who had been herded into RFK Stadium in Washington on May Day 1970 had been awarded money for the time the Washington, D.C., Police Department had deprived them of their civil rights. The inmates at Walpole could likewise argue that they were entitled to payment for the loss of their constitutional and civil rights to adequate health care.

Meanwhile, the Department of Correction prepared its own case. At this time, it hired Jay Harness, M.D., to be an expert witness. Harness, a surgeon at the University of Michigan Medical School and Hospital, had been the leader of a group that successfully turned around the abysmal medical care system in the Michigan state prisons. In the process, he became a national figure, perhaps the most prominent authority on prison health care. Word received by the Department of Correction had it, furthermore, that he thought everything was fine in the Massachusetts prisons and would say so in court. Because he was considered to be such a powerful and persuasive witness, the Department of Correction planned to base much of its case on his opinions. In 1985, Dr. Harness told Prout that he had indeed found deficiencies in the health care at Walpole and had so informed the Department of Correction.

THE CASE

Attorneys for the plaintiffs, Scott Lewis and Arlene Marcus, made it clear that they would make every effort to avoid the usual state and local political alliances that had stymied earlier efforts to reform health care in the prisons of Massachusetts by taking their case to federal court. Judge W. Arthur Garrity presided. Lewis wrote, in his pretrial brief to Judge Garrity:

> In 1971 the DOC [Department of Correction], DPH Department of Public Health], and DMH [Department of Mental Health] were advised by the Report of the Medical Advisory Committee on State Prisons (the Madoff Report) of the existence of serious systemic deficiencies in the delivery of medical care to inmates at MCI, Walpole. From 1972 through 1974, the DOC, DPH, and DMH were advised by the Prison Health Project of the continuance of those systemic deficiencies in the delivery of medical care to inmates at MCI, Walpole. From 1971 through the commencement of this action in 1977, the DOC, DPH, and DMH were repeatedly advised by inmates at MCI, Walpole, by the medical staffs at MCI, Walpole, and MCI, Norfolk, and by other departmental agents and employees, of the persistence of those systemic deficiencies in the delivery of medical care to inmates at MCI, Walpole. Since the commencement of this action in 1977, the DOC, DPH, and DMH have repeatedly been advised of the failings of the MCI, Walpole, medical care delivery system. In the fall of 1978, the DOC conducted a self-assessment survey and found many deviations from national standards in the policies and procedures of the Division of Health Services. In January 1979, the DOC employed a consultant to survey the state of health care services within the DOC; he reported systemic deficiencies in the delivery of health care to inmates at MCI, Walpole. In the spring of 1979, the DOC conducted another self-assessment survey and found substantial deviations from national standards in the operations of the MCI, Walpole, medical department. (*Alston et al.* v. *Hogan et al.*, U.S. District Court, Civil Action No. 77-3519-G)

During the summer of 1979, Judge Garrity approved the pretrial order and entered deadlines for the legal counsel to submit relevant materials. If Lewis could prove the assertions in his pretrial brief, Judge Garrity would give the inmates an injunction.

Meanwhile, the Department of Correction argued that the suit was no longer relevant. The damage case was gone and the injunction case was moot, they said, because they had already made great changes in the health care system. The Department of Correction, moreover, argued that they had plans for still greater improvements to the system. From the point of view of the Department of Correction, going forward with the injunction case was a waste of time. Nobody was then complaining about lapses in their medical care, they said.

Lewis and Marcus, their staffs and consultants, had spent much time on the case, and still they felt that they had only just begun their work. "We made the decision that their factual assumption that the system was working correctly was only marginally true," said Lewis. "Some things obviously were working a lot better than they had been. But there were still many holes in the system. More important, we were convinced that having our law suit pending had a lot to do with the improvements that had occurred. We did not want to relieve the pressure on the Department of Correction at that point. There was still much too far to go."

Judge Garrity, like Marcus and Lewis, understood that a suit like the Walpole case could go on forever, bogged down in endless details. Consequently, he pressed the plaintiff's legal counsel and the Department of Correction to agree first on the basic facts of the case. He was unwilling, he said, to sit through endless fights over the details of what did or did not occur. This was a difficult phase of the case. The Department of Correction was naturally unwilling to open its records to Lewis and staff. "It took an enormous amount of intervention by the judge to get the Department to do this," said Lewis. The Department of Correction tried to bury the case in the details; the plaintiffs and the judge tried to keep clear the outline of the argument.

Before the trial, counsel for the plaintiffs submitted a list of about two hundred exhibits and the Department of Correction submitted a list of more than one thousand exhibits. After examining the DOC list, Lewis felt that many of the documents listed simply did not relate to the Walpole case. "One was a nursing protocol from the Shirley prerelease center. It was clear as a bell that they had not done any work at all on the case," according to Lewis. "I went back to the judge and, in an extraordinary motion, I asked him to strike from the Court's record this list of documents the state was going to use. It was clearly unconsidered and irrelevant. He did. 'Unless you come up with a better list,' he said, 'you're not going to have any trial.' "

Lewis and his assistant spent almost all of their time for four months during the fall of 1979 sitting across a conference table from each other, debating the documents and facts in the case. They paid attention to the smallest details. What eventually came out of this tedious work was an important public document—a Stipulation of Facts, containing more than nine hundred paragraphs concerning the medical system at MCI, Walpole. The Stipulation of Facts contains the key documents generated over the prior decade relating to the issue of health care in Walpole Prison.

In summary, too, the Stipulation of Facts announced the major themes of the case and its remedy:

The plaintiffs and the defendants Berman, DiSimone, Ponte, Goldberg, and McNulty, for themselves and their successors, agents, and employees, stipulate for the purposes of this case only that the DOC has adopted and implemented, and that the DOC shall hereafter follow and maintain the following policies or practices at MCI, Walpole:

• Fully licensed physicians by contract with outside medical provider or medial group;

• Medical director or staff physician for "each inmate who is referred by paramedic . . . medical staff members or who requests to be seen by a physician for examination or treatment";

• No more traffic of incoming or outgoing inmates through the HSU;

• Daily records of treatment and drugs;

• Access to specialty clinics (amputee, arthrogram, arthritis, asthma, audiology, bone scan, brace, cardiology, convulsive disorders, diabetes, dermatology, dialysis, echogram, EEG, EKG, EMG, ENT, GI, hematology, medical, memory, neurology, nuclear medicine, occupa-

tional therapy, oncology, optometry, orthopedics, out-patient surgery, physical therapy, plastic surgery, podiatry, pulmonary, radiology, renal, speech, surgical, urology, and vascular;
- Arrangements with hospital to provide at least ten inpatient beds for exclusive use by inmates of state correctional institutions and arrangements with New England Medical Center, Massachusetts General Hospital, Brigham and Women's Hospital, and Beth Israel Hospital, on a rotation basis, to provide beds as needed;
- Dental services provided. (*Alston et al.* v. *Hogan et al.*, U.S. District Court, Civil Action No. 77-3519-G)

When Lewis and colleagues filed their pretrial brief, they established the structure of the entire case. Judge Garrity endowed the plaintiff's presentation of the case with greater authority by taking that structure as the model for the entire presentation. Over the vigorous protestations of the Department of Correction legal staff, Judge Garrity ordered the department to file its own pretrial brief under the same headings as that of the plaintiffs. This was a very important moment; the burden of proof was now shifted to the Department of Correction.

LEGAL REMEDY

Then came the endless negotiations with the Department of Correction, Department of Public Health, and the Department of Mental Health over details of the remedial orders. The Department of Public Health protested that they were just about to promulgate their own set of health regulations—the standards that had been called for in the statute of 1911. The Department of Mental Health, likewise, asserted that they were about to establish a system for upgrading mental health care in prisons. Neither department offered great resistance to the suit for remedial action.

But the suit asked the Department of Correction to spend money—at least $1 million a year to reform their health services. The remedy would indeed prove to be an expensive one for them. Nevertheless, by April 1980, lawyers for the plaintiffs and defendants came to agreement on what the judge's order should say.

The document hammered out in these negotiations was in effect, if not technically, a consent decree of a court of equity which allowed for alterations in its execution and allowed for supervision and enforcement to assure the rights of both parties. A successful simple lawsuit against a correctional department could find fault and assess penalties or damages, but such a suit would not allow for later modifications, inspections, or enforcement. This court would not be finished with the case on reaching a decision but would function, in some ways, as an executor or administrative agency. Naturally, this was a procedure upsetting to local courts, legislators, and politicians.

The document had two important characteristics. First, there were many detailed provisions concerning the medical care system, with specific dates by which time clearly specified remedial actions were to be taken. In seventy-two paragraphs, the statement went from peer review and setting staffing levels to requiring the promulgation of rules and regulations for all sorts of procedures.

Further, the document provided that after a few years, there would be a hearing to determine whether the Department of Correction had complied with all the provisions of the order. If the court found substantial compliance with the order, the case would be dismissed. If, however, the court found that there had not been substantial compliance with the order, the court was in a position to take any remedial action it deemed proper. This decision is a landmark in setting and enforcing prison health standards.

To get a feel for the strong language of the order, take, for example, the directive concerning segregated units: Within ten days of the order, the Department of Mental Health is to be provided by the Department of Correction with a list of all currently segregated units. Within three months, the Department of Correction will provide the Department of Mental Health with "written procedures for the provision of periodic medical and psychiatric examinations and indicated medical and psychiatric treatment to inmates in segregated units." The Department of Mental Health will review these written procedures, "stating separately for each proposed procedure whether it is approved, and if not, how it must be changed to obtain approval." The Department of Correction will supply a list to the Department of

Mental Health of psychiatrists and physicians responsible for providing medical and psychiatric care to inmates in segregated units. The Department of Correction will supply to the Department of Mental Health the name of each inmate confined to a segregated unit for any time during the preceding month, name and number, dates he received medical or psychiatric examination or treatment, and the type of treatment received. At least twice each year, the Department of Mental Health shall inspect MCI, Walpole, "and determine whether the Department of Correction has achieved and maintained compliance with the Department of Mental Health's protocols and has given adequate periodical medical and psychiatric examinations and indicated medical and psychiatric treatment to inmates in segregated units. The first inspection shall be made by September 30, 1981."

Similar orders were issued for monitoring and enforcing compliance with regulations "establising minimum health and sanitation standards and inspection procedures for correctional facilities and detention centers."

The Department of Correction was also instructed to prepare, adopt, and implement "a comprehensive policy and procedure manual for the provision of health services." This manual shall include, but not be limited to, description of the correctional facilities involved, goals of the health services program, organizational framework of the health services program, policies, and especially "policies confirming and defining the right of access to health care, the right to refuse treatment or participation in medical research, and the need for informed consent" for all medical procedures.

The details of the order repeat, almost precisely at times, the standards for health care in prisons developed by the NCCHC, based on the earlier work by the Prison Health Project, American Bar Association (ABA), American Public Health Association (APHA), National Sheriffs' Association (NSA), and finally, the American Medical Association (AMA). These include, for example, regulations for medical as opposed to administrative segregation, regular detailed medical supervision of segregated prisoners, health and sanitation procedures, a detailed policy manual, emergency procedures, and regular monitoring of all aspects of the health care system.

Thus, some seven years after the proposals made by reform-minded workers in the optimistic, but unrealistic mood of the 1960s and early 1970s, a workable and detailed systematic plan emerged. The judge's order seemed at last to have settled the issue, but the established bureaucrats and politicians had not given up. There are many tricks in the bag of a Massachusetts politician, as we shall see.

At Walpole there is a section that has been called variously over the years the "hospital," "infirmary," "Health Services Unit block," "HSU," or the "hospital block." The Health Services Unit at Walpole (which has inpatient and outpatient units) is a small L-shaped area off one of the main corridors. At the end of the Health Services Unit are fourteen cells intended for ill prisoners, which can be reached only by going through the medical unit. From 1975 to 1980, the fourteen cells were used as regular housing for inmates, presumably on orders from the administration to relieve the serious overcrowding problems. That meant that inmates passed through the Health Services Unit throughout the day, disrupting the medical system and compromising confidentiality. Worse yet, with the fourteen cells in the hospital occupied by healthy inmates, there was no cell to hold the sick ones.

To make matters still worse, underneath the hospital unit is an area known as the New Man Section, connected to the infirmary by a door and a set of stairs. In the original planning, new men were to be brought into Walpole through the New Man Section, and held until medical staff could perform the initial screening examination, before moving them elsewhere in the prison.

The New Man Section itself was an inhumane place without adequate air or light. The situation was so bad, in fact, that a federal court was already trying to shut down the New Man Section when the Walpole suit was being organized. To move new men meant bringing them up the stairs from the New Man Section and through the Health Services Unit, resulting in a constant stream of disruptive, unscreened, and unruly men passing through the health unit.

Scott Lewis argued during the litigation that not only was the block not being used for medical purposes, but also it was being used as a segregated unit, which, by regulation, must be supervised by the Department of Mental Health. This one was not, and it is doubtful if this consideration had even arisen at the Department of Correction.

In addition, all medical experts had for years strongly urged that this space be reserved for the medical department and that admission to those fourteen cells be solely decided by the medical director and for strictly medical reasons. In 1972 and 1973, the Prison Health Project had vehemently and repeatedly recommended that the fourteen cells be used solely as an infirmary. In the following years, others physicians echoed this request. When Dr. Ronald Goldberg took charge of health services at Walpole in 1978, he wrote a series of memoranda to the Department of Correction saying that he needed an infirmary. Finally, in 1979, before the consent decree was entered, the department issued a regulation establishing the fourteen cells as an infirmary, to which inmates could be admitted only with the approval of the medical director.

Even then, it was clear that the block was not being used properly. The prison census had grown to at least one hundred more men than capacity. There was no place for people to go. As late as the fall of 1982, there were still seventy people in the cells of the infirmary and in the New Man Section. There were double bunks in all fourteen cells, double bunks down the center of the corridor, and then mattresses on the floor between the doors to the cells. Downstairs in the New Man Section, there were about twenty-five people on the floor in an area marked off by chainlink fencing.

The correctional authorities were caught in an impossible bind. The courts ordered them to take this huge overflow into custody; another court was saying that human caring must be carried out. In this context, the requirements of custody and punishment clearly overruled the needs of caring.

There was no disagreement about the facts. Lewis went to Judge Garrity with the information saying that the order had been violated. "I'm not talking about whether the pharmacy regulations are precisely in accord with the AMA regulation. I'm talking about the fact that we have 70 people living in the hospital. That alone," Lewis reported, "constitutes substantial non-compliance."

The effort to clean up Walpole did not take place in a political vacuum. Prisoners are not constituents in the political system. They are not a voting bloc and they have no strong body of supporters among the enfranchised public. Nonetheless, politicians have a great deal to say about the correctional system. Political hay has been made out of law-and-order campaigns, escapes, riots, supposed coddling of prisoners, and, of course, out of the budgets for building, staffing, and maintaining houses of detention.

After agreement on the consent decree, many Massachusetts legislators becamse increasingly upset because many of the provisions were going to cost great sums of money. It came as no surprise to followers of Massachusetts politics that after the case between the Department of Correction and the plaintiffs at Walpole was settled through the court under Judge Garrity, the case was unsettled by the Massachusetts Legislature and by the administration.

There was a statute in Massachusetts known at the time of the consent decree as Section 39. This reflected the concern of the state legislature that bureaucrats of the state government's executive branch were entering into agreements that would eventually require the expenditure of large amounts of state funds. Appropriating and then spending funds was supposed to be under the control of the state legislature. Section 39 therefore provided that the commissioners did not have authority to settle cases without prior approval of the secretary of administration and finance. Section 39 called for thirty days prior notice to the chairmen of the House and Senate Ways and Means Committees, who could then overturn the entire consent decree with a legislative veto. The secretary of administration vetoed the Walpole settlement under Section 39. The agreement was rendered null and void.

"We went to court again in May 1980," said Scott Lewis. "I got up and Judge Garrity said, 'What's going on?' and I said, 'Well, a very interesting development. We reported to you that the case was over. It turns out that we have no agreement at all.' "

As Lewis was talking to Judge Garrity, he was considering the two things he might do next. He could ask the judge to make inquiry as to why the agreement was being abrogated or he could ask the judge to bring the case to trial. At trial, Lewis thought, he could offer the stipulated exhibits, call experts, ask the judge to enter as the injunction order the consent decree that the experts and lawyers for the Department of Correction had already agreed upon. Since it was already a matter of record that the Department of Correction had agreed to the consent decree, the trial would be a brief one. The consent decree would then become a compulsory order.

While Lewis was revolving these various points of strategy in his mind, Judge Garrity turned to the attorney general and said, "Mr. Gray, I would like to have Secretary Hanley come to Court tomorrow and explain to me what his reasons are for reversing the deliberate decision of the Commissioner of Correction. There are two ways we could go. It might be easier for all concerned if you would ask him to Court tomorrow at two o'clock or my clerk could call him." When the attorney general refused to ask Commissioner Hanley to appear in court, Judge Garrity replied, "Mr. Gray, there is a third alternative. I can instruct the United States marshal to arrest him bodily and bring him to Court tomorrow at two o'clock." "Perhaps I'll call him," the attorney general replied.

The following morning, Secretary Hanley delivered a letter approving the settlement with the Department of Correction. But then he rescinded his approval for the Departments of Mental Health and Public Health, only to be forced, once again by Judge Garrity to reapprove the agreement.

By 8 July 1980, Judge Garrity approved four orders: separate orders to three departments and a fourth stipulation that the Department of Correction was already doing the things the suit and Judge Garrity's order required of them. In Lewis's words, "Things were suddenly calm."

MECHANISM FOR LASTING CHANGE

The Walpole case had succeeded where the Prison Health Project had failed principally because it had had a Judge Garrity, a Scott Lewis, and a strictly defined legal mechanism that had not existed earlier for bringing about change and ensuring that the change would continue with deliberate speed.

As appears in all emotionally charged reform efforts, the Walpole lawsuit began to lose its vitality with the passage of time. The energy for it has obviously dissipated, but, more important, the plaintiff population has changed. Few of the original group of inmates remain in Walpole. The new inmates have not yet developed the rapport with the legal agencies enjoyed by the first generation of plaintiffs. Perhaps the inmates of today are not motivated by the same political forces as those of a decade ago.

The Department of Correction told the judge that there were plans to close the New Man Section, in any event. Consequently, the judge said he would do nothing. When in 1980 it was clear that men were still being housed in the New Man Section, the judge refused to reconsider. His decision was eventually reversed by the First Circuit Court of Appeals, which argued that the men who did not spread the feces on the walls had to be protected from the violation of their civil rights by those men who did. This is to say that the state must care for those whom other prisoners punish—a new twist on the paradox of caring while punishing.

After another period of negotiations, Judge Garrity issued another order forcing the Department of Correction to follow the letter of the original consent decree and order. In this instance, the issue of care being separated from punishment was relatively clear-cut, although in many details contested. When the punishment is inflicted by the inmates themselves, it becomes difficult indeed to decide for whom the state is obligated to take care.

These struggles caused the participants to lose sight of the goal: humane and effective health care for prisoners. The facts are clear and have been beyond dispute. Clear remedies were laid out in 1973 and earlier. The enabling legal and administrative framework had long existed. By 1981, two or three energetic lawyers and a hard-working and imaginative judge seemed on the verge of the success that had eluded so many others in improving prison medical services.

Three years later, there was less optimism. The public pressed the legislature and judiciary to put more people into prison. The Department of Correction was forced to house the much increased population of inmates, but the Massachusetts legislature would not give the Department of Corrrection the space or money with which to build and maintain the facilities they needed. The Department of Correction was, in effect, forced to defy the consent decree and agreement, in other words, to break the law.

Humane health care for prisoners clearly stands low in the hierarchy of what must be done. At a deeper level, consciously or unconsciously, many people seem to feel that prisoners are bad people whose suffering and privation are deserved. The division of powers and responsibilities in the Massachusetts system makes inaction possible, even likely. No one is satisfied with the present system, but no one feels he is at fault, either.

In 1978, the Department of Correction made a profound change in the structure of medical care at Walpole. They hired Ronald Goldberg, M.D., an energetic radiologist with strong entrepreneurial skills, to operate the medical system at Walpole with a medical staff he hired from outside the state system.

Goldberg was an independent contractor with whom the Department of Correction drew up a legal business agreement for the delivery of medical services. Over the next few years, Goldberg received and used more money than had ever been allotted to the prison medical system to hire physicians and to establish an elaborate medical and management system.

He came to Walpole in the fall of 1978, and by March 1979 he was also running the medical system at the adjacent Norfolk Prison. By the summer of 1980, "a watershed period in the case," according to Lewis, Goldberg had taken over all the institutions of any consequence in the Department of Correction. As a result, within three years of filing the law suit, the entire structure of the medical care system in the Department of Correction had changed.

The confluence of many factors eventually led to the overhaul of the health delivery system in the Massachusetts prisons. Without a doubt, the suit and threat of further litigation jogged the Department of Correction into action, but times had changed, as well. The general feeling of wanting to do good for the prisoners that had so ambiguously motivated the Prison Health Project just a few years earlier was replaced by a more sober and realistic desire for responsible budgeting, strict managerial accounting, and executive responsibility.

Alfred DiSimone, Director of Health Services at the Department of Correction, a longtime employee of the Department of Correction, was instrumental in directing this transition of the prison medical system. It is as much because of DiSimone's efforts as because of the threat of legal action that the system was so remarkably changed for the better. DiSimone feels that the transition to contract medical care has made his work easier and the care itself better. He says that from 1979 to 1986, although some 120 prisoners brought suit, the Prison Health Services Division did not lose a single case.

Since 1980, the Department of Correction's Health Services, under Ronald Golberg, has become a highly organized—some would say bureaucratized—system. Scott Lewis and associates continue to monitor the system from the outside, looking at documents from the Department of Correction, reviewing complaints from inmates at Walpole, and doing whatever is necessary to see that the system continues to satisfy the requirements established in the judge's orders. Complaints have been fewer and less strident.

4
Contract Health Care in Prisons

Providing health care to prisoners was originally a small part of the responsibility of the local authorities, who administered justice swiftly and arbitrarily. In America until the early nineteenth century, convicted felons or public nuisances were generally housed by the sheriff, who was paid a capitation or flat fee. This old arrangement is now once again coming to the fore in contract health care. Senator Arlen Specter of Pennsylvania has described an increasing trend for privatization of medical care in federal prisons as "the major unexamined new social policy of the 1980s."

At present, responsibility for medical care within prison walls is nearly everywhere in the hands of a department of correction. The medical care systems established by these departments vary with the type of prison, type of prisoner, local level of care, and above all with variations in official attitudes toward the medical care of prisoners. The size of the institution and its proximity to major medical centers affect the type of health care system. Often the various attitudes represent the influence of strong reformers or outstanding prison physicians—an influence that rarely, if ever, outlasts the reformers.

The welfare state philosophy of having various governmental agencies take total responsibility for the homeless, poor, disadvantaged, and imprisoned is being replaced, apparently with strong popular and legislative support, by contracting out care to for-profit agencies. Many hospitals in the United States are now operated by for-profit corporations. Some are wholly owned by private investors. It was only a matter of time before entrepre-

neurs offered proposals to operate entire prison systems on a
contractual basis.

Throughout medicine in the world outside prisons, free enterprise and what we might call the industrialization of medicine are
on the ascendancy. With the advent of such federal programs as
Medicare and Medicaid, health care became big business—approximately $400 billion annually in the United States. Attracted by
these huge sums of money, the Hospital Corporation of America,
Humana, and several others have organized highly profitable
health care organizations. Now, for a variety of economic and
political reasons, a growing number of for-profit companies are
offering health services just as any other service industry would
compete in the marketplace. In a 1983 Criminal Justice Institute
survey, 22 percent of the state correctional agencies in the
United States responded that they would consider contracting
the management of their entire correctional facility to an outside
firm; 74 percent would absolutely not consider contracting out
management; 4 percent were undecided. Kentucky and Pennsylvania were in the vanguard of this movement away from public
administration of correctional facilities.

The prospect of large budgets and commensurate profits has
brought into the prison management field such mammoth corporations as RCA, Control Data, Merrill-Lynch, E.F. Hutton, and
Shearson-Lehman. Under their offerings, investors become private owners of public prisons. Investors get tax write-offs, tax
shelters, and even profits as the holding companies lease their
prison properties back to the public. For example, the Corrections Corporation of America, based in Nashville, began running
a 350-prisoner work farm at Silverdale Detention Center in Silverdale, Hamilton County, Tennessee, in October 1984, on a contract of more than $8 million.

Privatization has made few inroads into state adult correctional
systems but has already had an impact on the federal system. For
a long time, privatization has been the preferred model in the
juvenile system. The most immediate prospect for private enterprise in the correctional setting is for community-based facilities
(for example, halfway houses and prerelease centers) where

there is a growing demand and a pressing need for a quick (and therefore not bureaucratic) response.

As of 1984, in eight states the private sector was involved in thirteen types of prison industries operated by departments of correction, manufacturing many types of products for private firms. In addition, there were privately managed prison industries not operated by the departments of corrections (in Florida, Oregon, Minnesota, Michigan, and Kansas) and privately managed federal, state, and local prisons and jails. As in so many other aspects of imprisonment, history seems to repeat itself. This ignorance of history arises, perhaps, because the burnout and turnover rate of people who work in corrections is so high. For example, when Chief Justice Warren Burger led a "new" crusade to "build prisons that are factories with fences" in order to return prisoners to society as "producers" rather than "predators," he repeated ideas of the British prison reformers, John Howard and Jeremy Bentham, who made similar proposals two centuries years ago.

Yet, according to one study, there is a surprising lack of information available on the processes and outcomes of contracting for human service delivery. "Assessment of the differences between public and private management are largely anecdotal: distinctions made between private non-profit and private for-profit contractors are also highly speculative." In general, however, the report concludes, "It is quite feasible to contract successfully for both traditional and technological functions as well as more intangible social products" (Mullen et al., 1985).

If medical care is viewed strictly as a necessary maintenance service, along with food, cleaning, light, and heating, then the philosphical objections to contracting out private medical care would indeed be fewer. As Mullen and colleagues point out, "Correctional facilities represent a powerful exercise of state power, as they are the means used to deprive persons in custody of liberties otherwise granted to all citizens (the most notable of which is freedom of movement). The delegation of this authority to private providers raises issues not encountered in contracting for more mundane services such as bus transportation and solid waste disposal."

PRIVATIZATION

We have seen that the medical care of prisoners is an issue fraught with social, ethical, and medical dilemmas and paradoxes. We can add to these the most interesting *economic* paradox that, on the one hand, states and municipalities complain that they cannot afford to provide adequate services to inmates of jails and prisons, and on the other hand, a private, for-profit enterprise (the Corrections Corporation of America) can offer $250 million to the state of Tennessee for a ninety-nine-year lease to run the entire state correctional system. Entrepreneurs and investors apparently see a gold mine where legislators and their accountants see only a bottomless pit. How can this be?

There is nothing unique about privatization of prison services. Public functions have been subcontracted to private firms in the past. Trash removal, fire protection, public safety, and other public functions are not always carried out by public employees. Today, because of the great interest in reducing public costs, we see a growing trend to turn to private enterprise for public service. Conservatives like the idea of privatization because it promises to reduce the size and scope of government and supposedly is more efficient.

Jails are not popular. Voters and the legislators they elect see jails and prisons as necessary evils to be supported at a barely adequate level but not with enough enthusiasm to allow significant innovations in correctional programs or facilities. Politicians are reluctant to appropriate public funds for prisons and jails and voters repeatedly reject bond issues for public works. Free enterprise has stepped into the breach. Representative Ray Keller, chairman of the Texas House Law Enforcement Committee, has been quoted as saying that privatization of prisons is inevitable in Texas "because while Texans don't like high taxes, they want criminals behind bars."

In short, the time has come for what has been called, in a typical Madison Avenue euphemism, "confinement service contracting." Private enterprise is now building prisons, staffing and operating them under contract with the state. These contracts, of course, include medical care along with security, food, transportation, and maintenance of the physical plant. One of the most dramatic changes in the correctional system brought about by privatization is the increased professionalism it introduces to a field not previously known for its high status and esprit de corps.

It is ironic indeed that the case work approach to corrections championed by such liberal-minded superintendents as Howard Gill and Miriam Van Waters may, in fact, finally become acceptable to legislators and others more or less interested in jails. Thus the liberal approach comes wrapped in the cloak of a professional contract between the state and hired caretakers. At the semantic level at any rate, relationships between the prisoners, guards, and doctors have changed significantly. At the Silverdale Detention Center near Chattanooga, Tennessee, the warden is called a "facility administrator," the guards are called "resident supervisors," and the prisoners are "clients:" Cynics can argue that, call him what you will, a "resident supervisor" is still a "bull" or "screw" and his "client" is still a con behind bars. This is true. But, regardless of the present realities of the matter, the intention to treat prison inmates as clients bespeaks a desire on the part of prison personnel to raise their own professional status, seemingly to the benefit of everyone.

Putting the job of prison construction out for bids has been promoted as the quickest and ostensibly the most inexpensive way to get a prison built. Private firms now entering the prison business maintain that they can build and run prisons at a cost at least 15 percent below that of public agencies. They attribute these economies to their use of more imaginative techniques and their avoiding the bureaucratic red tape in which governments inevitably get entangled. The Corrections Corporation of America has contracted to run the Hamilton County, Tennessee, prison at a cost of $21 per prisoner per day, $3 per inmate per day lower than what the county had been paying.

Encouraged by such cost projections, the nation's governors (as reported in the New York *Times*, 2 March 1986) have been increasingly in favor of putting prisons under private management to ease the problems of overcrowding and to reduce costs. In 41 of 50 states, departments of correction use at least one privately contracted service: medical/psychiatric (33 states), food

(21 states), security (4 states), transportation (14 states), maintenance (14 states), staff or inmate training (10 states), and others (7 states). The most commonly contracted are medical/psychiatric and food services, which are also the largest services.

No governmental agency can abrogate its ultimate responsibility for the well-being of its wards. Nor can any system, regardless of how well conceived it is, make a silk purse out of a sow's ear. In prison medicine, there will always be friction between a mistrustful and conniving group of patients, on the one hand, and perhaps inadequately trained and inadequately supported physicians and nurses, on the other. No health system can rise much above the mediocrity of the people running it; but a strong system, following established standards, well administered, can unquestionably improve medical care.

In addition to the possibility of reducing cost, one of the chief attractions of contract medical care in jails and prisons is the possibility of increased and regular supervision of the health care personnel. Supervision is one of the most important—and least appreciated—elements of a good health system. During a two-week crisis in 1973, for example, medical duties at the Walpole maximum-security prison were carried out entirely by residents from the Peter Bent Brigham Hospital, a large Harvard-affiliated teaching hospital in Boston. After the crisis had been resolved, these residents indicated in a questionnaire survey that they had found their experience to be highly unsatisfactory. It has become clear from their experience (and the experience of many others) that physicians, no matter how bright and experienced in general medical care, cannot function satisfactorily and cannot be persuaded to stay in prison work unless they can be assured of working under a stable medical system. Stability in this case means tight security, good records, a full-time experienced administrator in charge of the medical system, adequate paramedical help, and sufficient supervision to prevent the isolation and burnout that too often make prison work so difficult.

In February 1985, the National Institute of Justice convened a three-day conference on corrections and the private sector. After much discussion, the conclusion was reached that privatization is "a potentially attractive" alternative to public support. Privatization of corrections is supposed to be an efficient way to get the job done. But although many legislatures are at least considering contracting out the construction, staffing, and maintenance of their facilities to private enterprise firms, early results show that free enterprise may be no bargain either. The experience at Silverdale, Tennessee, is an instructive example. At the end of the first year, the cost overrun was $200,000.

The concept is old but the application of the concept in the present economic and political environment is too new to allow a thorough examination of its strengths and weaknesses. Experience will show whether entrepreneurs, inmates, or politicians will co-opt the system.

OPTIONS FOR HEALTH CARE

Poor management is historically one of the chief deficiencies of prison medical systems. For example, the simple failure to spell out precise lines of responsibility and standards of practice is commonly the basis of litigation. Health care and administrative personnel must each understand the legal and practical limitations of the other's position. Because of the poor communication and blurred lines of responsibility that characterize most departments of correction, however, each usually defines the responsibilities of the other only by bitter experience, and usually after conflict.

Management, like politics, is the art of the possible. There are very few, if any, absolutes. Consequently, in devising ways in which to manage prison medical systems, designers are immediately faced with a range of legitimate options, none of which is ultimately the best, but some of which are certainly better than the others. No management system is inherently better than another; each is better or worse suited to the practicalities and peculiarities of the setting in which it must operate. In short, responsibility for the medical care of prisoners can be distributed in several different ways.

The simplest and most commonly applied model is to have a department of correction take full responsibility for staffing and running the prison health care system. In this case, the medical staff and management are all state employees. Private contractual, for-profit systems can also be organized to assume responsibility for running the entire state prison health care system. In Arizona, for example, the entire state correctional system is subcontracted so that infirmary and other health care staff (as well as guards and food service) are employees of private firms under contract to provide goods and services to the state.

In a third model, as in Massachusetts, private employees under contract and state employees under public salary may work side by side in the correctional institutions. Contracts may be made with individuals as well as with subcontracting firms.

The simplest model is not always the most effective. Having the same employer—in this case, the state—responsible for direct health care, management of health services, security, and corrections creates serious problems by effectively removing the checks and balances by which all complex organizations are kept accountable. In the Walpole case, for example, the Massachusetts Department of Correction was part of the problem.

Increasingly, departments of correction throughout the United States have hired overseers of the health services from outside the correctional system. The successes of the accreditation programs conceived by the AMA and run by the NCCHC and ACA, for example, and the powerful influence of the courts have given ample evidence of the need to separate the functions of care and punishment.

The traditional operation of health units by departments of correction has been under heavy attack in recent years. As a result of surveys in state, county, and municipal systems, many reports, particularly in the optimistic days of the 1970s, advised separating the responsibility of medical care from the others of the departments of correction. To date, the problems raised by such division of responsibilities have been too great for most correctional systems. New York City and San Francisco are notable exceptions in their success.

It is obvious to us that separating a division of health care from the rest of the department of correction is absolutely essential, as is providing it with its own identifiable budget and a full-time director. The division can then contract out part or all of the health services while retaining ultimate control, a method that has been found to be effective in Massachusetts and other state and federal facilities.

Several health organizations present attractive alternatives to leaving health care in the hands of corrections: the department of public health, a large teaching hospital, a large nonteaching hospital, a medical care foundation, or a health maintenance organization; each may have the expertise and staff to run and manage the prison health care system.

Departments of public health have often been assigned responsibility for prison health care. This arrangement has substantial advantages but the disadvantages are even greater. For some years, the United States Public Health Service supplied the professional personnel to the federal prison system because from 1950 to 1972 physicians under the age of fifty were subject to the draft. A term in the Public Health Service was preferable for many to service in the armed forces. For this reason, the supply of physicians was adequate for the federal prison system. Before the draft, the Great Depression had made a salaried, secure position sufficiently attractive so that the Public Health Service had no great difficulty recruiting and keeping competent physicians and helpers. With the growth of medicine as a lucrative industry, however, salaried positions with the Public Health Service became less attractive. Physicians have been attracted by the high incomes available in private practice. During this drain of physicians away from public health work, the prison population has grown. As a result, fewer competent health professionals are available to treat a larger population of patients, so there is a clear shortage of health workers in the prison system.

Now new social and economic factors are changing the practice of medicine yet again. Medical schools have been training larger and larger numbers of physicians so that, at least in the most attractive areas, there is a glut of physicians. In most fields of medicine, too, incomes have stabilized and the risks of private practice are beginning to undermine the rewards. Consequently, secure salaried positions are becoming attractive again.

The advantages of public health departments' participation in the prison health system are their potential for recruiting and screening physician and nurse applicants, for surveillance of ongoing operations, and for epidemiologic studies and technical assistance, particularly in dealing with tuberculosis, hepatitis, AIDS in prisons, the control of venereal disease, and preventive medicine. Departments of public health, however, are not the solution to health care problems in prisons. In the United States at present, these departments are generally disengaging themselves from the delivery of direct medical care. The disappearance of tuberculosis as a long-term disease requiring hospitalization, traditionally a responsibility of public health departments, has much to do with this change. The trend in public health is toward systems, regulations, health education, and special epidemiologic and statistical work. In general, physicians and nurses working in the fields of public health have an orientation toward these specialized approaches and are often not interested in or temperamentally suited for actually delivering health care. Many of them have inadequate clinical training. As a result, fewer clinically oriented health workers enter the field of public health. San Francisco is a notable exception. The large and well-funded jail health program there is operated by a department of public health and has been successful in recruiting highly qualified personnel.

On the other hand, there are significant disadvantages in having a department of public health in charge of medical care in the prisons. In such cases, without changes in the laws, the prison superintendent continues to be in charge of the system operated by the department of public health. The superintendent would still determine personnel policy and would have the power to hire and fire the health personnel as long as security takes precedence over care.

Large teaching hospitals are capable of becoming ideal operators of prison medical care systems. The much-admired contract between the City of New York and Montefiore Hospital brings the experience and expertise offered by the large teaching hospital to all phases of acute and chronic surgical and medical care in large jails. The hospital also has a large staff so that rotation of personnel, so necessary in prison health work, is possible. The young and experimentally minded house staff can bring fresh approaches to prison medical care and specialty consultation is more readily available when needed.

There are problems, however, with the contractual arrangement between jails and large teaching hospitals. The staff of large teaching hospitals are by no means inherently possessed of the temperament and training needed in a prison physician or nurse. Continuity of medical care and knowledge of the individual inmate-patient's idiosyncracies are impossible if the entire staff is rapidly changing. If rotation through the prison system is a required part of an internship or residency, moreover, it is often accepted grudgingly so that the duties may be carried out in a perfunctory manner. Where large prison medical systems are successful, it is largely because of the wisdom and experience of a stable nursing staff. Furthermore, economy is uppermost in the minds of those who fund our correctional systems. It is well known that for all of its advantages, a teaching hospital is the most expensive health care facility.

The good reasons for the added expense of large teaching hospitals are that they are sites of time-consuming research and teaching as well as care; the physicians order many tests and X-rays. Critics argue, legitimately, that contracting with a major research and teaching hospital to provide routine care to a largely healthy population is unnecessary.

On the other hand, the economic position of large teaching hospitals is also changing, and for the worse. Funds have been cut back from many sources so that teaching hospitals, like all other hospitals, are looking for new markets. Hospital marketing in the community, industry, and even in the jails has become one means of keeping hospitals solvent.

Teaching hospitals, as the example of Montefiore shows, can do the job well. Such a plan needs a full-time prison medical administrator trained in prison work and a full-time physician with similar orientation. The problem with such an arrangement, however, is that ultimate hiring, firing, and security clearance remain legally under the department of correction. It is an open question how much of this responsibility a department of correction can delegate to the hospital.

Many features of using the teaching hospital as operator apply to a nonteaching general hospital as well. Nonteaching hospitals also may have a large, well trained staff, but the recruiting of staff members to deliver prison medical care is difficult since no valuable training or other tangible benefits are offered. Appeals for help remain personal and emotional. There is a potential advantage in having available mature, experienced physicians, particularly those with general practice training and experience. The type of physician who will agree to work with prisoners usually has a strong background of community involvement. It goes without saying that the medical staff should be well paid and, again, that there should be a full-time administrator to act as liaison between the hospital and the correctional facility.

The most rapidly developing trend in medical care delivery in America lies in the health maintenance organization (HMO), either nonprofit or for-profit. To many legislators and correctional authorities, to be able to hand over all responsibilities for prison health care to an outside agency provides a welcome relief from an unpopular and uncongenial duty. The HMOs or medical care foundations consist of groups of physicians and other health professionals whose members have agreed to work on a retainer or fixed fee-for-service basis. They work together under a set of well-defined regulations, with a large administrative superstructure and varying types of reimbursement for the physician. The earliest successful HMOs were the Health Insurance Plan of Greater New York and the Kaiser-Permanente Foundation on the West Coast. Now such organizations are everywhere.

Theoretical advantages of contracting out such care to an HMO are that medical care can be delivered in a variety of large and small institutions, urban and rural, without placing too heavy a load on any one physician or group, and reimbursement is assured by contracting organizations. Also, medical care of the inmate could be continued by the same professionals after the patient is released from prison or while on furlough. If integrated into a medical care system for the inmates' families, the result might be a more humane, effective, and economical form of health care. Unfortunately, to date, no HMO has put such a plan into effect with complete success.

Most recently, there are organizations designed specifically to provide health care to jails and prisons on a contractual basis. In effect, these are medical groups paid by a third party outside the department of correction to provide services to jails and prisons. The appeal of such a system to the federal, state, or municipal departments of correction is that they pay a predictable, fixed, and budgetable amount. Because it is buying a year's worth of care, and not paying for treatment episode by episode, the department of correction can call for bids or bargain over the price and allegedly get more service for less money.

PROS AND CONS OF MANAGED CARE

The for-profit, private firms maintain that their programs are better than public programs because they are cost-effective, allow greater quality control, make the contracting firm more accountable than the public employees, improve efficiency, and increase flexibility. By the simple calculus of free-enterprise economics, the argument goes, the contracting party first wants the contract (low cost) and then wants to keep it (high performance) at a profit (high efficiency). By establishing a centralized management and budget system, the firms promise to make the system cost-effective. Because they are accountable to an outside organization, they may protect the corrrectional health system from litigation. By providing contracts on open bidding according to requests for proposal (RFP) that are widely distributed, they supposedly assure the public that the programs eventually set up will meet certain health care standards while saving the public money.

In addition to the clear economic attractiveness of the contract care approach, there are other less tangible advantages. The first and most obvious appeal—and it may indeed be a great advantage to the health care team—is that interposing a layer of non-governmental administration between the prisoner and the state helps to a certain extent to divorce care from punishment. The operation of correctional health care in Westchester County, N.Y., is an example of one successful arrangement. Dr. Allan H. Rappaport, president of National Emergency Services, which operates in the western United States, has written, "If the doctor professionally carries forth the medical duties oblivious to the fact that the patient is an inmate, then he can render appropriate medical care compassionately without prejudice or the appearance of taking sides" (personal communication, March 1984). This officially neutral attitude parallels the statements made by Professor and Dean Norval Morris of the University of Chicago Law School to the effect that if the health care team follows precisely the laws, regulations, and standards that have been well laid out, doing neither more nor less than is required, then they have created the "best" system.

The second advantage is that the contract arrangement helps prevent that common occupational hazard of prison medicine, burnout. Competent and aware contracting entrepreneurs can rotate staff and indoctrinate able "moonlighting" health care professionals. Human nature being what it is, it seems to us from personal experience that it is almost impossible to work in a prison sick line or visit a prison infirmary without having strong emotional reactions, usually a variety of conflicting reactions. In isolation, physicians and nurses faced with the emotional rigors of working in the correctional setting eventually either become so inured to the difficulties that they lose their ability to function as empathic healers or, just as bad, they become increasingly sensitive to the peculiar demands of their work and cease to function adequately as objective workers.

Affiliation with the department of correction, in some ways, increases their sense of isolation and alienation from the rest of the medical community. Affiliation with a for-profit enterprise, rather than directly with a department of correction, can remedy some of these problems for the physician and nurse. There can be a greater sense of professional worth, it is easier to arrange for peer review, and the physician or nurse is not so isolated from the rest of the medical community.

The motivations of health care deliverers and of corrections officers have traditionally been suspect. Physicians who work for the correctional system, whatever their qualifications and motivations, are assumed to be working in prisons because no one else wants them. Why so many fine nurses continue to work in prisons is not so clear.

In the past, this suspicion might have been justified; but in the present medical marketplace, the overproduction of physicians is changing employment patterns. Young physicians are eagerly seeking salaried positions in HMOs and other contractual relationships rather than opening their own offices. As a result, the caliber of physicians and nurses in prison medicine has risen significantly. They are professionals seeking to do professional work, with all the professional supports afforded other physicians in other settings. In fact, there is some talk of organizing a subspecialty to be known as the American Academy of Physicians for the Incarcerated.

Contract health care is no panacea either. There are significant disadvantages to contracting health care out to for-profit firms. "Going private" always raises the apparent budget for health care. As advocates of privatization are quick to point out, however, this increase in the medical budget is offset by savings in the higher quality of the health care given to prison inmates, by the easier access to specialty clinics, by the reduced absenteeism and down time of staff and facilities, by the more flexible use of medical resources, and most important of all, by the reduced likelihood of litigation.

Going private does require far more complex relationships between the clinical and administrative personnel of the health care and the corrections offices. When these work well, however, they increase the appropriate supervision of health care personnel, create the mechanisms for centralized resolution of conflicts, and establish coherent and strong standards of professional conduct throughout the health care system. For advocates of privatization, these advantages are worth the added costs of increased bureaucratic control.

A stronger objection to contracting out prison health care is that it seems to most people to be fundamentally wrong in some vague and unspecified way. The threat of privatization to the civil service and the labor unions is clear. The American Federation of State, County, and Municipal Employees (AFSCME), for example, opposes the private operation of prisons and jails, fearing that the 40,000 present prison guards will lose their jobs. But there is a more difficult and pervasive feeling that making a private profit from a public responsibility is somehow indecent. Why the moral stature of civil servants is higher than that of other people working under contract, however, has not been explained.

To recapitulate, we see some good in contract care, but it is not the ultimate solution to the problems of bringing adequate and affordable medical treatment into jails and prisons. It is simply one of several possible means, although it is one that satisfies the present social and political urge to reduce the size and influence of government.

The advantages of contract medical care, under strict supervision, are the possibilities for flexibility, ability to try new modalities of treatment, responsiveness to new situations, and the ability to transfer personnel from one area to another in cases of unusual need.

As stated by one contracting firm, the goals are to: reduce the number of complaints and sick calls; reduce the prescribing of controlled substances; reduce the need for transferring patients from one type of health care facility to another; and reduce the cost of administrative details. Each of these goals is two-edged, however. For simply to *reduce* services may cut costs, but avoids the much more difficult questions about how much to cut while still providing adequate medical care.

How much to reduce the number of complaints and visits to the sick line will always be an unanswered question. In one year reported, one inmate in three visited the federal health facility in Leavenworth on a given day. Seen as a strictly management problem, such overutilization of health care resources is costly and inefficient. Having a large part of the inmate population show up daily for sick call may actually produce secondary gains—for the prison as well as for the inmates. The inmates clearly can benefit from the attention they get from sympathetic nurses and physicians. The prison as a whole, too, may benefit from the truce established by satisfying the almost insatiable need for attention on the part of some inmates. On the other hands, in most jurisdictions, the inmate may sign a form indicating that he or she chooses to refuse treatment. This refusal can be interpreted to include the costly initial physical assessment. In at least one for-profit prison health system (judging from admittedly anecdotal evidence), the inmates are not discouraged from signing this form.

Access to medical care is a loaded emotional issue for inmates who have a lot of time to think about their own physical and emotional states, who crave opportunities to test the system, and who feel isolated and alienated from normal, safe human contact. In the prison uprisings of the 1970s, access to medical attention took on symbolic value at least as great as that of the straightforward health concerns of the inmates. Regardless of the initial causes of the riots in Attica and elsewhere, the tangible and publicly appealing issues of access to medical care became the rallying cry as the riot progressed and as the prison conflict became an issue in the news media. In the management battles of the 1980s, health services may again take on such symbolic significance. It is a gross oversimplification to think that physicians must see only sick people and that seeing healthy people on sick line is an abuse of the system. The job of the health care team, rather, is to differentiate between the sick and the well, to treat the sick, and to reassure the well. Cutting the sick line to some low number by administrative fiat is therefore not necessarily practicing effective medicine in the prison setting. Moreover, increasing the anxiety levels of the inmates deprived of access to what they perceive as needed medical attention can only have adverse effects on the prison environment.

The second goal, reducing the prescribing of controlled substances, is good only if it is the result of a medical rather than a management decision. Reducing all medication is a reasonable goal only if the reduction is consistent with the practice of good medicine.

The third goal, reducing the need for transferring inmate patients from one type of health care facility to another is also a mixed good. If the number of transfers is reduced because specialty facilities are available under one roof, the reduction is all to the good. If, however, the reduction in transfers comes when a powerful gatekeeper says no to keep costs down, except in the most pressing cases, this runs against good medical practice, common decency, and ultimately against fiscal good sense.

The fourth goal is to reduce the amount of administrative detail. As yet we do not know whether centralization is cheaper or more effective. The real relationship between reducing administrative detail through centralized organization of health care and reducing administrative costs remains to be studied adequately.

The final goal of meeting the standards of the American Correctional Association and the National Commission for Correctional Health Care is the most promising of them all, for that would institutionalize the oversight of health care in prisons and jails, a powerful argument for the for-profit model of health care. Because they pay the malpractice insurance, the contractors have a vested interest in keeping good records and delivering good medical care while relieving the prison physician of the ever-present fear of malpractice suits. In Massachusetts and in other states, prison physicians have been severely damaged by malpractice judgments in which the state either did not reimburse them or reimbursed them only slowly and in part.

ETHICAL CONCERNS ABOUT THE PLACE OF PRIVATE ENTERPRISE

John Maynard Keynes once remarked that capitalism is the extraordinary belief that the nastiest of men, for the nastiest of motives, will somehow work for the benefit of all. The American suspicion of politicians and entrenched civil servants is only matched by naive faith in the purity of the free enterprise system. In corrections, as in many other areas of American life, a system based on competition and profit is expected to succeed where systems based on governmental power have failed.

Questions about the place of private enterprise in connection with imprisonment are typified by a remark by Mark A. Cuniff, executive director of the National Association of Criminal Justice Planners: "We are talking about taking people's liberties and I have a real question about the propriety of anyone but the state doing that." The introduction of for-profit contractual arrangements to build and run prisons raises profound ethical issues that are sure to inflame the emotions of almost anyone who considers the subject in detail.

An article in the *New York Times* (17 September 1985) summarizes the possible adverse effects of private control of prisons: (1) pressure for longer sentences, (2) reduced use of halfway houses and probation, (3) reduced alternatives to incarceration, (4) lobbying abuses, and (5) public relations campaigns to convince the American population of the dangers of crime.

The most important considerations, of course, are those regarding the quality of care and the cost. In prison medicine as in most other fields of medicine, the balance of cost and benefit is delicate and difficult to compute with any assurance. Students of medical economics have been trying by various methods in an enormous number of ways to measure the quality and cost of health care in general. By any measure, there is no clear verdict at this time as to what is a fair return of health care for the dollar and whether the for-profit sector is any more efficient or effective than the not-for-profit sector. The question of costs cannot be settled because it is virtually impossible to find suitably comparable groups.

Beyond the difficult questions of economic feasibility, there are the broader questions of policy and ethics in the for-profit operation of prison health care. The primary question is obviously that of the propriety of the whole idea. Have we as a society violated our own basic concepts of public responsibilities by contracting out the care of our prisoners? When the prison physician is paid by the Department of Correction to care for the inmate population, the client is the inmate. When the care of inmates is given over to physicians and other health professionals under contract to outside private enterprise, the community is the client and the incentive for better care is economic rather than professional.

The contractor has a vested interest in hiring high-quality nurses and physicians. Pay and working conditions are therefore made competitive with those found outside prison medicine. Good care is provided to minimize the liability of jail health systems and to minimize the ultimate cost of caring for an inmate population.

On the other hand, there is the phenomenon that has come to be called "the Sheraton syndrome." Just as hotels are designed to be economically feasible at near-full occupancy, so hospitals must keep their beds full to avoid undue losses. Are prison health services that are run under contract to turn a profit for the investors and proprietors under similar pressure to keep the beds full, in a sense, by keeping as large a captive population as possible? Or, contrariwise, if they are paid a lump sum, do they want to keep the hospital empty, denying care to some who need it? The manipulations of census figures in some municipal hospitals and even in some V.A. hospitals comes to mind as useful reminders of how the health care system can be manipulated for profit.

There is a widespread interest in making the inmates pay, at least in part, for their room and board in prison. "For the most part, prison industries continue to labor under a variety of legal and administrative barriers that inhibit the widespread participation of free enterprise. At the same time, however, this area of private sector participation may hold the greatest promise for changing current confinement practices." The notion of a prison as a total worklike environment that might operate on a profitable basis, contribute to the costs of confinement, and provide useful training and productive work opportunities to confined inmates is an extremely appealing vision that has been widely discussed as a model for American prisons of the future.

Recent studies have cast serious doubt on the claim that private health care organizations run for profit (for example, HCA, Humana) may be operating at lower cost or greater efficiency than at first appeared. There is the phenomenon of dumping the patients with more serious and expensive and long-term illnesses who have no third-party insurance into public hospitals. Even the cost-effectiveness of treating a cross section of the population does not appear, according to the recent studies, to be better done in the for-profit than in the not-for-profit medical institutions. It is possible, for example, that contractors of medical care would arrange for the transfer of rebellious inmates whose attitudes were unsatisfactory and whose care was difficult and expensive. This recalls the complaint of Howard Gill's successor as superintendent of the Norfolk Prison that he was being sent difficult prisoners. These prisoners might be transferred to a state-run facility, relieving the private contractor of this burden.

Once again, we see that the health care of prisoners needs scrutiny. The more layers we peel off this onion, the more layers we find. Public accountability covers institutional inefficiency;

private efficiency overlies the desire for profit; all of them surround public sympathy, which, in turn, covers public fear of the convicted criminal. Beneath the fear is hostility. And still we are not at the core. It is difficult indeed to construct a rational health care system on the shifting sands of such powerful and unexamined emotions.

In actual fact, it seems to us that the state has already taken away the inmates' liberties and even has power over the ability and authority of private contracting organizations to preserve whatever liberties and rights the prisoners are still entitled to.

Part II
REALITIES AND LIMITS

5
The Prison Health Care Environment

Fear and boredom are the cardinal points of the inmates' emotional compass. Theirs is the fear of cornered animals turned desperate by the ever-present signs and symbols of their captivity. Short-term inmates may be driven to suicide by the isolation they feel and by their total reluctance to identify with the environment of which they find themselves captive. Long-term inmates, in contrast, usually manage to find a modus vivendi, a temporary truce with themselves and with the prison environment. It is the only way to survive.

Inmates may survive by adopting any of several basic strategies: (1) retreat into fantasy, (2) solidarity with the other inmates, (3) commitment to an ideology that gives meaning to their incarceration, and (4) opposition to authority (Cohen and Taylor, 1972). Regardless of the psychological defenses they adopt, however, inmates cannot wholly avoid the realities of the physical environment in which they find themselves. Nor can the prison personnel, for that matter. Short of frank psychosis, inmates and prison staff are faced with the unpleasant and unsatisfying task of living and working in an environment that is designed to be less than comfortable. In such an environment, the best they can hope for is sheer coping. The worst is unimaginable. For the convicted felon, one might say, this is the expected reward for antisocial behavior. What is one to say, however, for the health professional who more or less freely chooses to work in this setting?

Physicians treating inmates must be in the prison. The practi-

137

cal reasons for having physicians near their patient population are obvious. There are other more subtle reasons for putting physicians in the prison setting. In fact, the greater the privations in the prison, the sharper the need for a knowledgeable medical presence. Ignoring this simple fact has led to many sad errors of judgment.

In the general population, the American physician seldom makes the time-honored house call, and the resulting poor clinical information about the patient's environment has significantly changed the practice of medicine. Some would say that this has been a change for the worse. If the prison physician similarly ignored the environmental factors of prison life, the practice of medicine behind bars would be severely hobbled. To protect himself against the conniving and self-seeking inmates, the physician needs a strong ego, without question, and a clear sense of what the inmate's game is. Only firsthand experience of the prison setting can give him this kind of knowledge. In a more complex way, too, the physician must know the subtle deceits that are commonplace in the prison. Just as the inmates are likely to make much of nothing, in the interest of stirring up trouble or simply to get attention, so inmates are likely to withhold important medical information if they think that revealing it will put them in jeopardy. In either case, the prison physician must take the inmate's information with a great deal of skepticism. The only way to evaluate the reliability of what he is told, therefore, is to know the prison system as well as the inmate knows it.

John Cheever's novel, *Falconer*, captures the salient features of the prison environment: inescapable stress for inmates, guards, and health workers. Farragut, an educated man convicted of killing his brother, is brought to Falconer Jail, "this old iron place," built in 1871.

> Falconer was very shabby, and the shabbiness of the place—everything one saw and touched and smelled had the dimension of neglect—gave the impression, briefly, that this surely must be the twilight and the dying of enforced penance. . . . The bars had been enameled white many years ago, but the enamel had been worn back to iron at the chest level, where men instinctively held them. . . . But all of this, all that

there was to be seen and heard, was wasted on Farragut, who perceived nothing but paralysis and terror. (p. 4)

By their very nature, jails are places of deprivation. Inmates are deprived of freedom, association with loved ones and friends, movement, sex, choice of what to do and when, creature comforts, privacy, food, attractive scenery, and all the other large and small voluntary decisions that make life pleasurable. In addition, inmates live with the constant threat of violence, sexual assault, arbitrary or mistaken disciplinary action by guards, and every other possible imposition of power that can make life, in Hobbes's words, nasty and brutish. Finally, inmates are deprived of access to the drugs and alcohol to which most of them had been addicted before being admitted to the prison.

Anger, fear, hostility are inescapable in the large jail. No one is immune. Inmates most obviously suffer the indignities and intrusions of prison life.

Guards, of course, choose to work in jails and prisons; but, in time, even the most committed correctional officers feel somewhat trapped by their choice. As one guard has said to the authors, "Most inmates are eventually free to go. We stay." This sense of frustration, compounded by the ever-present resentment of the inmates and the poor support given corrections by the outside community, mounts to anger and hostility. Medical workers are yet another group frustrated by the prison environment. No less than the inmates and guards, most health workers in jails and prisons would rather be somewhere else.

The nature of prison aggravates the stereotyped antagonism between inmate and guard, according to Goffman. Forced loss of identity, recurrent indignities, and loss of privacy are part of the process of social control of the inmate. As in the earliest experiments in prison reform—the reformatory movement, the penitentiary movement, and other means of giving social and moral value to the simple fact of enforced solitude and incarceration—the modern inmate must learn the system and social code of the prison to earn the progressive privileges and eventual freedom. Throughout this process, the staff of the prison protects itself and preserves its own integrity by depersonalizing relationships with the inmates. Inmates, no less, maintain their emotional equilibrium in the bizarre world of the prison by alienating themselves from their environment and from the people around them—both inmates and guards.

Yet both the staff of the prison and the inmates also want to be liked. For guards this is an especially difficult problem. They need to feel that they are humane and kindly people, but in an environment so charged with the potential for violence, fear is a necessary and protective adaptation. The defense against fear, most often, is hostility.

Most guards speak of their concern for the welfare and feelings of the inmates under their supervision, and they are convinced of their own sincerity. At the same time, a guard will also say that he feels unappreciated and that if he is too compassionate he is likely to be exploited by the inmates. As a defense, the guard will say that this is not generally the case. Only some inmates would take advantage of a kind guard, but the guard must be constantly vigilant lest that exploitative inmate make a fool of him.

Nicholas Pileggi has described the uneasy truce between inmates and correctional officers in the New York City Prison on Riker's Island (*New York Magazine*, 8 June 1981). The prison, say correctional authorities, is "better ruled with a light touch than with a heavy hand." That means allowing the prison system to develop its own social organization, which Rikers Island has done, according to Pileggi: the top tiers and corridors, for instance, are usually reserved for drug use and homosexual encounters. Officers rarely encroach upon this inmate turf. The president of the Corrections Officers' Association described the place as "out of control."

> Officers are just not backed up. Inmates see they can still commit crimes and there is no deterrent. If they are found with drugs, they are not arrested. When visitors come in with weapons, the weapons are returned to the visitors when they leave. Everyone is conspiring to keep the lid on, and we're paying the price.
>
> A corrections department official in New York City says, "The system now works, but if the guards got greedy or the inmates felt they were hassled even more, I wouldn't want to be around for the

results. In a jail where inmates wander around all day long, can have sex, turn on, watch television, have contact visits with wives and girlfriends, get free magazines and papers, use law libraries, and where 125 meals are routinely cooked for every 100 inmates, there's little need to pay off anyone."

Take the simple example of attempting to maintain a drug-free or alcohol-free prison. Severe restrictions on contact between prisoners and visitors, rigorous searches of visitors, and frequent surprise searches of inmates and their cells by corrections officers cannot free a prison of drugs or alcohol. They will merely heighten the resentment of inmates, their families, friends, and civil liberties lawyers.

Alcohol is not only brought into the prison by many imaginative means but is sometimes even fermented or distilled within the institution itself. Drugs are brought into the prison, often in packages inserted into the natural openings of the body. Careful body searches would naturally severely curtail the flow of illicit drugs, but to conduct the searches with the degree of care necessary to find the contraband would be time-consuming, expensive, and legally dangerous since innocent visitors to prisons would be subjected to degrading and discomfiting searches of mouth, anus, vagina, clothing, and accessories.

As is the case in so many other aspects of prison management, what might be done cannot be done. The legal, medical, and administrative considerations of stopping the flow of contraband by means of strict body searches totally overrule the possibility. The result is a feckless policy against drugs and alcohol.

PHYSICAL REALITY: INTO THE PRISON

Usually the first impression of a prison or jail is its depressing, restrictive, and authoritarian atmosphere. The building is usually old, but age itself is not the problem. Some of the older prison buildings are actually better designed than the newer ones. Benjamin Henry Latrobe (1766–1820), for instance, was one of the great American proponents of the Greek Revival. He and his pupils constructed Greek Revival public buildings. Among these imposing and beautiful edifices are the Bank of Pennsylvania, the Bank of the United States, several government buildings in Washington, D.C., and the innovative prisons of Philadelphia. Likewise, Charles Bulfinch (1763–1844) designed public buildings in Boston, several state capitols, and the state prison in Charlestown, Massachusetts.

The ongoing debate over what to do with the Charles Street Jail (Suffolk County Jail) in Boston shows that we still honor the esthetic values on which those architects designed their prison houses. The Charles Street Jail was designed by J. F. Bryant Gridley and dedicated in 1851. Although the building has fallen into disrepair, efforts to demolish the imposing granite structure have been defeated. A deal with the neighboring Massachusetts General Hospital involves a land trade, relocation of the jail to a tract of land currently owned by the hospital, and an agreement to restore the old Charles Street Jail for another use.

In earlier times, architects could make more generous use of space, air, and light than they do today. With their basic facilities updated, these older buildings would be serviceable, indeed. However, although age and poor maintenance are not necessarily synonymous, they often do go together when the buildings are not venerated. Public buildings are often renovated to maintain their esthetic and historic value. Jails, it seems, are generally exempted from this consideration; the Charles Street Jail was a hard-won victory.

Many of the older jails and prisons, of course, were not designed by first-rate architects. In addition to the crust of age and poor maintenance, in the case of these buildings, shabbiness, forbidding cold stone, concrete, or brick, and the closeness of a castle keep make these buildings singularly unattractive. The lasting impression made by these older jails is one of stolidity.

The impression made by newer jails and prisons, however, is no more favorable: social utility achieved at the expense of human scale and humane values. Towering above inmates, guards, staff, and casual visitors are the high walls that surround most jails and prisons. Atop the wall are razor wire, barbed wire, or jagged pieces of broken glass. At the corners of the walls, guard towers dominate the scene. The sense of being watched, but watched by someone who cannot be perceived in turn, pervades the area during the day like the searchlight at night.

For the casual visitor, there is always discomfort. Finding a parking place is often difficult. The visitor approaches the door to the prison self-consciously and enters the reception area with trepidation. Around the reception area, doing official and unofficial business, it seems people are always waiting, making little attempt to camouflage their hostility. They are waiting for news, for a visiting pass, for permission to enter, for permission to leave, for permission for any of the myriad large and small acts that cannot be done by outsiders without permission. Often, after prolonged delays, permission still does not come. The custodial staff knows this and deals with the visitor in an intentionally impersonal manner.

The health worker is and is not part of this system. Even the giver of care must submit to the inevitable series of security checks. Physical inspection, passing through the sensitive metal detectors, close and sometimes hostile scrutiny by the custodial staff, requests by friends and relatives of inmates, doubts—all assail the health workers who approach the prison doors.

This is a new world.

Despite the press of people and the commonplace overcrowding of the living space within jails, the inmates and the people who watch over them are usually silent. After meals or at recreation time, however, there are occasional outbursts of talkativeness. Boredom may be responsible for much of the uncommunicativeness of the inmates. Mutual antipathy and distrust keep the inmates and guards from all but the most businesslike and perfunctory conversation.

Perhaps more important, inmates and guards alike must spend inordinate amounts of time and energy in the effort to maintain even a modicum of privacy. Usually the only sanctuary left is the inner world. Casual conversation is a needless intrusion on another's inner world and, by the same token, is a potentially disastrous extrusion of one's own. Then, too, inmates and their warders are sullen and angry people with little information or feelings to share easily. By far, silence is the better policy. Despite the press of humanity, the inner world of the prison is not a human world. In the absence of talk, the silence is punctuated by the sound of steel on steel. Doors clang shut. Shouted commands and reprimands echo down the corridors, amplified and distorted by the peculiar acoustics of concrete walls and steel bars. Only the smell of the prison is human. Stale tobacco smoke, poor ventilation, burned grease from cooking, inadequately flushed human excreta all contribute to the overpowering atmosphere of the prison. The sharp scent of antiseptic solutions betrays the futility of any gestures to lighten the atmosphere.

Unlike light outside the prison, inside it never seems to spread to fill the space. Shafts of light come in from outside, passing through skylights or narrow slits of windows. The glass is thick, reinforced with heavy wire, and is rarely washed, if ever. Inside the prison, bare light bulbs, shielded in wire cages, burn around the clock. Like the lights in a subway tunnel, they seem to burn but illuminate nothing.

High above the walls, the sky continues bright and clear. This is especially true of the larger prisons located outside the city in the more rural parts of the state. Within the walls of the prison, most facilities have an enclosed yard for exercise and recreation. The yard is often a place of poignant contrasts. The greater part of the field is covered with weedy grass that has been trampled by many feet. Bare patches blow dust in the dry weather and turn to mud in the wet. In the inaccessible corners of the yard, however, inmates may have planted and tended with loving care flower and vegetable gardens.

WHY MAXIMUM-SECURITY PRISONS ARE SO OFTEN IN THE COUNTRY

Most maximum-security prisons in the United States were built, in the nineteenth century, far from the unwholesome atmosphere of the city. The rationale at the time was to remove inmates from the unhealthy physical and moral influences that had led them to crime.

The stated intention was to build large, rural, symmetrical, fortress-like structures, emphasizing the strength, stability, and rationality of society and the structures it could build. Placing the prison in the midst of pristine natural beauty was somehow supposed to shore up the weakened moral supports of the criminal even though the prisoners could see none of the outer facade of the building and almost nothing of the countryside in which it was set.

After this theory of reform and correction was discredited and superseded by more "modern" psychological, sociological, and (now) physiological theories, the habit of putting prisons in the countryside did not die easily. Newer prisons are still designed with the criteria of the old.

To strip the cant from the accepted rationales, however, it is probably more accurate to say that the prisons were located far from the urban centers for several quite practical reasons: to transport inmates from their familiar surroundings; to put the unpleasant social realities of prisons out of sight and mind of the public; to build large institutions on cheaper land; to create jobs in economically depressed rural areas; and to avoid the inevitable objections of neighbors and real estate agencies to placing jails and prisons in areas where real estate was valuable.

There are, instead, serious operational disadvantages attached to putting the large prisons in such isolated settings. Attempts to organize medical care in prison systems make it abundantly clear that no prison should be isolated from the mainstream of the community. Isolation makes it virtually impossible to get good specialty and consulting care. Moreover, it is impossible to recruit regular trained health teams to work in professionally isolated settings. In simpler terms, if health workers in the prisons cannot take advantage of convenient public transportation, must live far from the amenities of urban or suburban life, cannot find adequate schools for their children, need to drive ten or fifteen miles to find a supermarket, and so on, the chances of finding dedicated professionals to work on the health teams are significantly reduced.

HEALTH AND SANITATION

The American Bar Association standards recommends that prisoners be provided with a "healthful" place to live with quarters allowing "substantial privacy," freedom from excessive noise, and protection from disease, property loss or damage, and protection from personal abuse. "Every correctional institution should comply with health, sanitation, fire, and industrial safety codes applicable to private residential facilities or public buildings" (American Bar Association and American Medical Association, 1973).

No one would disagree with such a statement, but building new prisons costs vast amounts of money. Nevertheless, at least fifty new prisons are currently proposed or planned in the United States to provide an additional 25,000 beds, at costs ranging from $35,000 per cell to more than $65,000. That is a total cost of from $875 million to well over $1 billion.

For obvious reasons, the construction of prisons is controlled by the criminal justice system. Design decisions are primarily governed by the needs for security. Suggestions from the medical team are sorely needed as new prison facilities are designed and built, but recommendations about environmental health or the design of medical facilities have rarely been solicited. The allocation of space, control of sound, light, ventilation, location, and a host of other health-related design and construction issues are usually handled by adapting the state and local building codes to the peculiar requirements of security. As a result, the design of new prison buildings is most often a compromise.

Compromise is not always the best policy, however, for in designing structures as specialized as large prisons, research and experience often show the clear superiority of some design strategies over others. One important factor needing special control, for instance, is sound. At times, the interior of a prison is deathly still; at other times it is painfully loud with strident voices and the clangor of steel on steel. At all times, the sound inside the jail or prison is unnatural. The science of psychoacoustics is still in its early stages, yet it is obvious that the peculiarities of sound level and sound character inside the prison have significant psychological—and even physiological—effects. During a violent disturbance, for example, the noise is a major part of the event itself.

Even moderately loud sounds, if they continue long enough—

and certainly shorter bursts of extremely loud sounds—can impair hearing. The United States Environmental Protection Agency (EPA) has defined eighty-five decibels as the maximum acceptable sound level for industrial settings. No one is charged with the responsibility of testing the sound levels in prisons. More subtle and less easily defined adverse effects of excessive noise include feelings of nervous tension, the tendency to startle more easily, and an increased sense of discomfort and annoyance. Inmates in prisons are usually already tense and angry. The constant bombardment of sound merely heightens their unpleasant hypervigilance.

Loudness is not the only consideration. Pitch, how often the noise occurs, and the content of the noise are also important. Intermittent noise, for example, is more disturbing than constant noise at a fixed level. The unexpected and uncontrollable aspects of noise are most painful and unsettling.

Noise spreads. Prisons are typically built of stone and concrete, with steel walls, doors, and bars. There is little or no sound-absorbing material on the floors, walls, or ceilings. Furthermore, because of the peculiar acoustics of the prison setting and because of the characteristics of the inmates and guards, people tend to talk loudly. As the sound level in the prison rises, naturally people find that they need to speak even louder. Again the sound level rises. Shouting is contagious. During a violent confrontation, moreover, the sound level rises even higher, fueled by the angry and hostile feelings of the participants and onlookers. Acoustic engineering to damp the sounds of the prison might help cool the situation. A bit of quiet would certainly help keep observers, health workers, and corrections officers a bit cooler, as well, as they recognize the unmistakable signs of a riot atmosphere growing and spreading.

Light is another important design factor. Too much or too little light can be profoundly disturbing. Prisoners of war, for instance, have been broken by being confined in a room with constant bright or dim light. Too much unshielded light in hospitals, likewise, has been shown to disorient the workers and patients. When intensive care units in hospitals learned to modulate the light, differentiating night from day, anxiety and disorientation of patients were significantly reduced.

Ventilation is always a problem when large groups of people are confined in a relatively small, enclosed space. It makes little difference if the group is the audience in a concert hall or the inmates in a large jail. Airborne infections, unpleasant levels of humidity in the air, and the many subtle and not-so-subtle body odors of the human animal are all concentrated unless the ventilation system can efficiently remove them. In the older prisons, the ventilation system simply recirculates the air. The system does not have an efficient intake for fresh air or a vent to the outside to remove stale air. Instead, the hundreds or even thousands of inmates of the prison breathe and re-breathe the same sea of air and its increasing freight of airborne contaminants.

Overcrowding of jails and prisons in the United States is becoming a major public issue. Crowding is potentially dangerous from a public health and mental health perspective. Close crowding of inmates may be responsible for the spread of the many communicable diseases affecting human beings. Beyond this, crowding large numbers of angry prisoners—most of them men—into small spaces increases the likelihood of serious group violence.

Paradoxically, undercrowding as well can be a potent source of stress on prison inmates. A prisoner may be separated from others and confined by himself in a special isolation cell, usually for one of three reasons. *Solitary confinement* is a particular form of punishment meted out by correctional authorities much as a stern parent might banish a wayward child to his room. *Segregation* is another form of isolation in which the inmate is separated from the other inmates for his own protection. Finally, *isolation* may be a therapeutic intervention, for medical or psychological reasons.

The psychological effects of all forms of isolation may be powerful. Isolation, even for the most benign therapeutic reasons, often imposes hardships on the inmate. In a social system such as that of the prison, where most people try to survive by attracting as little attention as possible, isolation, separation, and selection for special treatment of any kind must carry with it the potential for reprisals. The use of segregation is emotionally charged because the inmate is already threatened by inmates or other members of the correctional institution. In the paranoid system of the prison, even segregation for one's own good may make the segregated inmate all the more vulnerable.

The most psychologically trying form of isolation, however, is solitary confinement. This is a sometimes brutal form of punishment ordered by correctional authorities as an extreme punishment or as a means of protecting guards or other inmates from violence threatened by the inmate.

The psychological effects of solitary confinement are harmful. They are meant to be. For most health professionals called upon to supervise the progress of solitary confinement, the experience is painful and highly objectionable. The physician, nurse, psychologist, or medic may find witnessing that form of punishment painful. In time, the health professionals may find themselves opposing the correctional authorities. When solitary confinement produces severe reactions in isolated inmates, the demands of the health professionals and the requirements of the correctional authorities come into direct conflict. Nevertheless, solitary confinement remains a reality of prison life. The "hole" or the "bing" may be the only permissible form of punishment available to correctional authorities.

Most correctional authorities impose solitary confinement reluctantly. They often feel anxious or even guilty about punishing inmates by such blatant shows of power. When health professionals criticize or question the use of solitary confinement, however, correctional authorities may respond with defensiveness and anger and, as a consequence, become more intransigent. The careful medical professional learns, in time, to approach the issue with tact and circumspection lest he find that despite his best intentions he has worsened the situation.

Because of the special physical and mental stresses imposed by solitary confinement, the health care team might be consulted whenever this form of punishment is imposed. Health care professionals might also be consulted in the design of solitary confinement cells, as well. Most cells are poorly lighted and poorly ventilated in the belief that solitary confinement is a punishment and should therefore be as unpleasant as possible. Nevertheless, depriving an inmate of adequate light and air contravenes constitutional and statutory protections against cruel and unusual punishment. The solitary cell, like any other cell in a correctional facility, must be large enough, ventilated adequately, and sufficiently lighted to qualify as humane treatment.

The use of solitary confinement cells for the purposes of medical segregation and isolation compounds the problems, for often the inmate is punished by the very process of protecting him. Suicidal inmates, for example, may be segregated from the rest of the prison population in solitary cells. Private space may be reassuring and sedative. Moving an agitated inmate from the normally crowded conditions of the prison to a more sparsely populated area often calms him.

The use of solitary confinement cells as therapeutic environments, however, is questionable. The shielded light fixtures, nonflammable bedding, and specially designed protective plumbing of the solitary confinement cell make it a perfect isolation cell for suicidal inmates. The rigors of unsupervised solitary confinement, however, the unpleasantness of the physical environment, and the sense of isolation and alienation from the rest of the prison community may very well exacerbate the emotional turmoil of an upset inmate.

Cells in general should provide enough space to be comfortable. Confining men in space of less than eight square meters per person doubles the incidence of social and physical pathologies. Privacy is important, at least for part of the day. For some inmates, companionship is also important and reassuring. Authorities in Bristol, England, found that when crowding conditions required that prisoners be placed two to a cell, the incidence of violent behavior and suicide attempts dropped dramatically. Most new prisons are now built with one-man cells. One knowledgeable and experienced observer, Joseph Rowan, formerly of the National Commission for Correctional Health Care, feels that this practice, in direct conflict with experience, will increase the suicide rate among inmates.

SOCIAL REALITY: PEOPLE OF THE PRISON

In this physical space the people of the prison live and work. Inmates, in complex and paradoxical ways, are the clients of the system. Administrators and guards, kitchen staff, and medical staff are the providers of services, also in some complex paradoxical way, to the clients. But unlike most provider-client relationships, this one is a grudging one, on both sides.

Guards

In official parlance, guards are *correctional officers* but to virtually everyone who works or lives in jails, they are *guards* or referred to by other even less complimentary terms. Unlike the benign and bureaucratic neutrality of the phrase *correctional officer*, the term *guard* connotes power of one person over another, heightened security of the institution, and strict control of inmates' behavior.

Throughout literature and history, guards and jailkeepers have been despised characters and they know it. To this day, many prison guards socialize only with their fellow guards. They do not boast of their occupation to others. Officers are often the sons and grandsons of officers, carrying on a family tradition that they probably would not have entered on their own. They are born to the work.

The very fact that the correctional system has tried to substitute these terms is instructive. Guards are watchful and protective. An officer, in contrast, is a holder of a public trust. The two functions overlap to some extent; but they are not identical. In trying to change the terms, the correctional system has attempted, at the very least, to elevate guards to the status of professionals. Until recently, however, educational requirements were minimal, and guards were often less articulate, less educated, less self-assured than their charges.

Little wonder that guards have been easily manipulated by inmates. Guards are subjected to the mixture of hostility and sociopathy generated by inmates. Not wanting to see themselves as bad people, guards must try to make some kind of peace with the inmates they watch over. Often this means identifying with the inmates. Because the general public either ignores or condemns the guard, identification with the inmates is all the easier.

As guards strengthen their bonds with the inmates, they are increasingly vulnerable to manipulation by them. "Whereas liberty engenders democratic thinking," writes Bruno Cormier, a psychiatrist who has worked for more than twenty years in Canadian and New York State prisons, "captivity produces paranoid thinking. . . . Constant exposure to paranoid thinking presents the danger of being drawn into it" (1975, p. 10).

The temptation to reach some kind of accommodation with the prisoners most readily takes the form of trading favors. Guards can guarantee themselves at least a modicum of peace or, in other circumstances, can amass large sums of money, by striking deals with the inmates.

The most successful prison guards have a genuine interest in their work and a real desire to serve the needs of the correctional system, on the one hand, and the requirements of their inmates, on the other. These guards know the social system of the prison—both the power structures established by the inmates for themselves and the political structures established by the administrators of the prison. They also recognize the social and political position of the prison in the larger society beyond the prison walls. Such a prison guard is rare indeed. When the medical team is blessed with the luck of having such a guard to work with, their own work is lightened.

Generally, however, prison medical staff run into problems with guards. The guards are inured to the problems of working with inmates but they are sensitive, perhaps overly sensitive, to the criticisms of outside professionals working inside the prison. New prison health workers are especially difficult. The do-gooder is universally disliked and distrusted. Although welcomed by the manipulative inmates of the prison, the amateur reformer is persona non grata among the professional prison workers.

But aside from the special case of the do-gooder, most physicians, nurses, and technicians working inside the prison are the object of corrections officers' ambivalent attitudes. The first reception is cautious. Then after a long period of testing, the health team and the correctional staff will usually reach an agreement and decide to work together. Without mutual accommodation, neither group can function in the prison setting and they are united by their resentment at the criticism and lack of support from the outside.

Even the best guards are changed by years of frustration, bitterness, rage, fear, and failure. Some guards become calloused. Many find relaxation and then escape in alcohol. Depression and apathy enervate them and make them ineffective as guards and as human beings. No statistics are available, but it is the distinct impression of many prison physicians that there is a high death rate from coronary artery disease among guards.

Guards burn out within a few years. This rapid turnover of correctional officers prohibits the continuity on which a coherent correctional policy must depend. Rules and regulations cannot succeed unless the personnel are in place to put them into action. If personnel are constantly changing, the institution soon forgets what has been done successfully, what policies ended in failure. Rapid turnover of personnel, too, prohibits friendships among the staff and positive relationships between staff and inmates. More like strangers than staff and clients, the cast of characters relentlessly changes.

Correctional staff come to the prisons by one of two routes. Wardens, superintendents, and guards may be appointed to their positions as part of the political patronage system on which any state or local government depends. In jails and houses of correction, the administrator is the sheriff, an official elected to office for reasons often independent of his competence, training, or special interest in criminal justice. Administrators of large prisons may have risen through the ranks, protected by civil service, or may have been appointed to their positions by virtue of their training in criminology, law, or sociology. The career corrections officers who have worked their way up the administrative ladders to positions of leadership are usually committed to the work and remain on the job. Highly trained appointees, in contrast, are more likely to move from one facility to another or even out of the corrections system entirely.

Health Workers

The chief hazard to the prison health worker is the profound effect of being exposed continually to so much paranoid thinking and hostility within the prison while not being adequately supported by people outside. The world within the prison takes on a separate reality, one divorced from the more familiar social, political, moral, and intellectual habits outside the prison.

Health workers have a singular advantage over other professionals who must work with prison inmates; the mission of the health worker is clear. Inmates may not understand or support the mission of the social worker, the occupational therapist, or even of the psychiatrist, but they certainly understand the roles and goals of the physician's assistant, nurse, or the physician. As a result, when the prison's social and physical environments make it possible for the health workers to carry out their functions, the job of providing adequate medical care to the inmates is not a difficult one. Difficulties are imposed by the peculiar conditions of the criminal justice system and by the special characteristics of the prison inmates.

Despite the many obvious disadvantages attached to being a prison health worker, many highly motivated and dedicated professionals work in the prisons. Few stay long; most leave in despair, with bitterness, anguish, and sadness. Melvin S. Heller (1974, p. 25) describes the situation:

> deprivation and political and bureaucratic craziness get the doctor. He can quit and get away. He usually does. What does he do if he stays at it? He stays a little longer time in the lunchroom. He smokes that second pack of cigarettes. He gets a big belly. He develops pet, slightly paranoid theories about life and people and especially prisoners. He becomes professionally more isolated and tends to go to fewer medical meetings because he doesn't see that much that his patients have in common with other patients. . . . The prison doctor working alone has a heavy responsibility, and has to serve time and live with his mistakes. So what's the alternative? I do not think, if I were a warden, that I would have the average physician working full time.

Self-discipline, self-knowledge, and maturity are absolute necessities for the job. It is impossible to see and talk with fellow human beings behind bars without being moved by their plight. Regardless of the heinousness of the crime, it is difficult not to sympathize with the person who has been deprived of so many of the simple rights and pleasures we take for granted. The successful and long-term health workers in prisons are mature, have realistic expectations of what they can and cannot do, have strong egos, and enjoy more than a little irrational selflessness.

Although the team approach is considered a liberal reform of medical care in general medical practice, within the prison system it is demanded by necessity. Time, money, speed of treatment, availability of personnel, and the many other particular conditions imposed on medical care within the walls of prisons and jails require a team approach.

Nurses

In the vast majority of jails and prisons, the leading members of the team in terms of time spent with the patient and knowledge of the system are the nurses. In 1972 the American Nursing Association became the first professional health organization in America to address officially the issue of improving medical care in prisons. Rena Murtha, R.N., to name just one active member, has been from the beginning an inspiring leader and one of the few who has maintained an interest in prison health care. The American Nursing Association has published an excellent manual for nurses working in jails and prisons. In the years since they have taken an active interest in prison medicine, nurses have assumed several roles within correctional systems: primary care; hospital nursing; mental health nursing; epidemiology and public health work; coordination of medical services; and serving as medical advocate for the inmate-patient; research worker; and health educator.

Nurses are, in fact, the backbone of the correctional health care system. In large organizations, a nurse may carry out no more than a single role. In smaller jails and prisons, one nurse must carry out all these functions.

Paramedics

The economics of prison health care and actual experience elsewhere show that good medical care can be delivered to large numbers of inmates by paramedical staff under the direct supervision of a single physician. Physician extenders or physician's assistants can multiply the effectiveness of a single physician. The medical needs in most prisons and jails in the United States are simple routine diagnosis, preparing and dispensing medications, and giving routine first aid for common injuries. Most of the time, a paramedic can provide just as good care as a fully trained physician. The proper use of physician extenders and assistants, therefore, in no way lowers the quality of medical care and actually raises the quality by freeing the physician to care for the more complicated medical cases.

There is a large reservoir of former military medical corpsmen in the United States, many of whom were trained in the Viet Nam War. For a variety of reasons, many of these well-trained men and women have been unable to find satisfactory work in the private sector and have found their way to work in the prisons. These former military medical corpsmen have been used in the Chicago jail health service, to name one system that has been studied carefully, where they have been rapidly accepted. In Massachusetts, where military corpsmen have been an important addition to the jail health program since 1972, they have significantly improved health care.

Physicians

People inside the prison wonder why the physician, who could make a good living on the outside, has decided to squander his life inside. Outside the prison, people wonder what was wrong with the physicians who chose to work inside the prison. The fact that the health worker may have taken the prison job voluntarily makes him doubly suspect. As we saw in the discussion of managed care, under contract, in the correctional setting (see chapter 4), the physician who works solely for the money is the only one whose motives are clearly understood and respected.

Until a few years ago, all prison physicians were true general practitioners. The prison doctor was expected to be all things for all occasions, embodying in the real world the myth that exists in our popular culture of the old-time American physician who could deliver a baby, set a broken bone, treat infectious diseases, and perform minor and major miracles by sheer intuition. Many of the best prison physicians have been persons of great personal strength, energy, and resourcefulness. The care they provided often compared favorably with that given to the average American citizen by the average American physician of fifty years ago.

Times have changed, however, so that medical care that would have been acceptable in the United States fifty years ago is no longer permissible in modern prisons. One indication of this change is the growing recognition of correctional medicine as an independent subspecialty. Today the health workers in prisons function as a team, with less emphasis on the physician as the sole and ever-present arbiter of diagnosis and treatment.

General qualifications for the good prison physician are difficult to describe. The most obvious characteristics of the good physician—excellent professional training, intellectual curiosity, sense of wonder and adventure, good communication skills, strong sense of justice and fairness, and the desire to help other people—have been shown by hard experience to be insufficient in most prison settings. Paradoxically, these virtues of the fine physician serving in a general practice serving normal middle-class patients may actually be counterproductive. Prison practice is just not that simple.

First, the question of authority. In any medical practice, the physician must sometimes tell patients to do unpleasant, unfamiliar, and painful things. However, in the outside world, the patients have chosen to be treated by him and by implication want to cooperate. Even in this best medical situation, however, patients are unlikely to adhere strictly to the regimen prescribed by the physician. Sometimes patients simply do not understand the instructions. At least as often, patients fail to follow instructions for a host of far more complex psychological reasons involving denial of disease and its effects. Compliance is always a problem: patients fail to take their medications according to the prescribed treatment plan, patients fail to maintain prescribed diets, or patients fail to get prescribed therapeutic equipment. In general practice, the physician can only assume that the patient recognizes the value of the prescription and, motivated by self-interest, will adhere to the prescribed course of treatment.

In the prison setting, in contrast to the general medical practice, the physician has infinitely more control over the patient; and, because the courts have found that the correctional system acts in loco parentis when it takes custody of an inmate, the physician also has far greater responsibility. At the same time, however, the physician is also confronted by an infinitely more recalcitrant patient.

The need to establish authority is obvious in dealing with prison inmates, yet no population is more unruly and sensitive to the imposition of discipline and limits. No physician or nurse can be effective for long if authority derives from simple dominance. Maturity and experience season the work of the best medical staff. Prison nurses, medical corpsmen, laboratory technicians, physician's assistants all must learn to command respect on terms established by the inmates, and this takes toughness.

A history of military service has proved to be an advantage for anyone working on the prison health team. The work environment in prisons is very much like that of the military. The sensitive idealist is vulnerable in the prison setting. The risk of disillusion is great. The realist, who looks directly at the great problems inherent in any attempt to bring adequate medical care to the prisons but resolves to do what he can, accomplishes the most in the long run.

In prisons as in the military, the medical team is dealing with a young, healthy, and principally male population. Medical conditions of the young and healthy predominate (as we will see in the next chapter): infectious diseases, trauma, and the effects of drug and alcohol dependency. Chronic or life-threatening conditions, characteristic of older populations, are relatively rare. As in a college student health service, military setting, or any other treatment of essentially healthy people, the rarity of serious disease nonetheless increases the risk. In the search for the needle in a haystack, medical staff may become less careful, not expecting to find illness.

Also as in the military, the prison health team must work within a strictly disciplined organization devoted to keeping its members under control. Outside the prison (and the military), the physician is often called upon to help the patient maximize the potential for human freedom. Inside the prison, the physician and health team work to help the inmate tolerate the rigid restrictions on his freedom.

Psychiatrists

Most prisons in the United States do not have the full-time services of a psychiatrist. Rather, a psychiatrist visits the prison regularly to carry out the necessary evaluations of emotionally troubled inmates, as well as to classify and treat emotional and psychological disorders. Most of the ongoing treatment of inmates is carried out by psychologists, social workers, general physicians, nurses, and medical corpsmen.

Forensic psychiatry is a special branch of psychiatry that deals with the legal aspects of mental health problems. If the correctional system were set up ideally, the forensic psychiatrist would concern himself only with the legal aspects of the inmate's mental condition—determinations of mental competence to stand trial, degree of criminal responsibility, assessment of legal considerations involved in transferring the inmate from one prison to another, supervision of the civil rights of the inmate, evaluation of the threat posed by the inmate to himself or others, determination of the need for legal services, regular review of the need to isolate certain prisoners. In fact, the psychiatrist is in an especially awkward position in a prison setting. Psychiatrists and mental health workers serve both the patient and the correctional system.

The prison psychiatrist treating the inmate must get the confidence of the inmate-patient, but the information he gleans is often of great legal importance. The psychiatrist treating the patient and the forensic psychiatrist serving the needs of the criminal justice system are often the same person.

PHYSICAL EXAMINATIONS

The initial physical examination of an inmate is a critical event. It may be the first careful checkup the inmate has ever received and it sets the tone for all subsequent relationships between the inmate and the medical team. In a larger social sense, it may introduce the inmate to the health care system outside the prison as well.

In the best prisons, new arrivals are kept in a separate section of the prison while being observed and classified. The examination is conducted in an atmosphere very different from that of a private physician's office. A guard is within earshot. Although the examination is required by law and custom, there are questions as to the extent the prisoner can refuse all or part of the procedure. In most instances, no one, for example, can be forced to submit to a rectal or vaginal examination without a court order. Yet in the setting of a private physician's office, such examinations are a normal part of the complete physical examination.

Within less than an hour of arriving at the prison, according to the American Medical Association standards, a correctional officer must make a brief notation of the prisoner's apparent health status. This is simply to note whether the prisoner is apparently healthy, conscious, rational, and free of complaints that might require emergency treatment. The correctional officer also notes such conditions as alcohol or drug intoxication.

A routine history and physical examination are frequently scheduled to take place within twenty-four hours of being admitted to the prison. But the AMA standards call for physical examination only within *fourteen days* of admission. The reason for this divergence in official opinion is that prisoners staying fewer than fourteen days are usually lost to the health care system, making the detailed physical examination and history a pointless waste of time and effort. Prisoners staying fourteen days are likely to stay in prison even longer so that the time spent on the examination and history is well spent.

Once prisoners have become part of the prison medical system, their usual point of contact with the medical staff is through the sick line. Establishing an orderly procedure for sick call, seeing patients under the sometimes adverse conditions of the infirmary, arranging and dispensing medicines, and notifying inmates of their medical status are all difficult within the constraints imposed by the prison or jail setting. Access to medical attention creates a problem; for although all inmates are legally entitled to medical attention, it is also well known that some prison inmates will try, for reasons of their own, to gain unlimited access to the system.

The larger the institution and the longer the sickline, the more impersonal the interchange between physician and patient. The

abuse of sick call at Leavenworth, as at most prisons, is probably
an effort to break down this impersonality. Heller points out that
"tender physical intimacy has been a rare luxury in the lives of
most prisoners. It is as though tender touching was interrupted
during their childhood at about the age of three. . . . Prison sick
call then should involve some touching, some warmth and humor
in response to the prisoner's request for medical attention in an
emotionally bleak and deprived atmosphere" (1974, p. 25).

In most prisons, the guard is the gatekeeper to the medical
system. Inmates must present themselves to the guard for permission to join sick call. Unfortunately, this practice gives the
guard undue disciplinary power by allowing him to grant or withhold permission to join sick call. The tradition of petitioning
through guards also puts medically untrained personnel in the
position of making sometimes subtle medical decisions.

The courts have struck down this practice, arguing that only
medical personnel are trained and competent to make the appropriate triage of patients. But the court decisions do not clarify
how the already overworked physician and nurse can perform the
necessary separation of the sick from the not-so-sick and the
healthy and, at the same time, examine and treat the bona fide
sick inmates.

For those who are unable, for reasons of disability, to come to
the sick line or who are being held in their cells in isolation,
seclusion, or segregation, in some institutions a sick call slip is
used to summon the physician to the patient. Breach of this practice is a serious infraction of the constitutional guarantee of medical care in prisons.

The system of sick call is designed to suit the needs of the staff
rather than those of the patient. Just as patients in open office
hours in a crowded physician's office, inmates are treated first
come, first served. These conditions, exacerbated by the crush of
inmates waiting to be seen and by the limited number of hours in
the day, lead to a quick and superficial appraisal of the inmate's
medical status. More serious problems are put off until after the
rush of sick call.

In all successful large prison medical systems, the initial contact, primary care, and evaluation of the inmates' health status

are all carried out by nurses, nurse's aides, or physician's assistants. These paraprofessional staff members are often better acquainted than the physician with the prison culture and the social network that forms such an important part of the inmates' lives.

Initial sorting of patients, screening, and emergency care are often better provided by prison nurses and experienced medical corpsmen than by fully trained physicians. Too often the physician who comes as a visitor remains aloof and ill at ease in the prison setting. In the tense world of prison medical emergencies and in the manipulative world of the sociopathic inmates, the distant and disengaged physician is both ineffective and likely to be conned. On the other hand, a good physician and team leader, having given sufficient instruction to the medical team, carefully supervising the work and acknowledging the invaluable assistance given by the team can assure inmates of the prison of completely acceptable round-the-clock medical care.

MEDICATIONS

In private practice, it may be enough for a physician to diagnose conditions and prescribe the appropriate medications. For the prison physician, this is only the beginning. The dispensing of medications is a major source of discontent, occasionally leading to riot as it did in Walpole Prison in 1972. At best it is always a problem.

A settled, firm, reasoned prescribing policy minimizes the chance for inmates to manipulate the medical system. Those prisons where the least medications are prescribed are those with the most manageable pill line and with the least harrassment of medical personnel. The new nurse, corpsman, pharmacist, or physician is invariably tested in the matter of prescribing and dispensing any drugs that have an effect on the central nervous system. Stimulants, tranquilizers, pain killers, and any other drugs that have noticeable effects on the senses are avidly sought—perhaps merely to break the tedium of long days in jail, perhaps for sale, perhaps to heighten the sensations of homosexual encounters.

Whatever the reasons, the search for drugs is unending and tireless. Easy marks are quickly identified. In the maximum-security prison at Walpole in 1972, after a period when there was no regular physician, many inmates gratuitously received daily doses of narcotics and hypnotics. Reestablishing orderly procedures involved tremendous effort and cooperation on the part of physicians, nurses, pharmacists, medics, and prison administrators. Even with these efforts, many months passed before a reasonable minimum of prescriptions could be achieved.

Prescribing policy can be relatively trouble-free if rules and policies are posted in the medical facility, in the pharmacy, and in the superintendent's office. According to the AMA standards, the number of days for which a prescription is valid is to be stated clearly. Prescriptions for hypnotics, narcotics, and sedatives are to be reviewed weekly. Prescriptions are to be written by physicians and dispensed by physicians, nurses, or pharmacists only.

Part of the problem is that personnel are not always available and the rules regulating how drugs are dispensed must be bent occasionally, if not broken entirely. If no one else is available to dispense medications, sometimes a guard or even an inmate must be given the responsibility even though this is against all accepted standards and even against the law.

This practice is fraught with danger because many medications have a high resale value in the prison culture. The dispensing inmate may steal the drugs or may give them to the patient in excess or reusable form. It is common practice in jails, for instance, to hold the pill or capsule in the cheek pouch, pretend to swallow it, and then on leaving the pill line, immediately remove it for sale or hoarding for later in larger doses. Dispensing medications in liquid form or as crushed pills makes this traffic in drugs impossible, but, as in the difficulties in Walpole Prison, the guards' practice of crushing all medications before giving them to inmates can bring about a major civil rights fight in the courts.

HEALTH CARE FACILITIES

No part of the American health care system excites more interest, controversy, or regulation than hospitals. This is even more true of hospitals for prisoners. To go to a hospital on the outside is to seek caring and intensive treatment not available or possible at home. Inside the prison, hospital care means the same things but also much more.

Prisoners, at least as much as other people, may be slightly hypochondriacal, bored, anxious about their health, or just in need of human compassion and contact. Outside the prison, people seek medical attention to satisfy many of these needs. Inside the prison, needs are even greater. Prisoners can see a trip to the hospital as a more than welcome change of locale. It may offer a much-sought chance to escape, to trade drugs or information, or to manipulate transfers to other prison facilities.

In the many surveys made of prison medical care in the United States, a comparison is made between the standards of care inside prison walls and those expected of an urban general hospital. The discrepancies, although recognized as obvious and necessary by several court decisions, are at the same time the basis for continuing litigation. A careful look at the situation makes it clear that in several respects, notably speed of medical response and the degree of privacy afforded the inmates, there is no way that a prison hospital can meet the standards of an urban general hospital. There are delays in treating emergencies in prison hospitals, confidentiality of medical records is often breached in the higher interests of security, privacy must be curtailed in a setting where inmates must be watched at all times, and access to people outside the prison, too, must be severely limited.

The range of prison facilities is from simple day care centers in the small urban jails or lockups to large, fully equipped and staffed general hospitals.

The simplest day room is an incomplete medical facility suitable for small institutions (fewer than 100 inmates) in which round-the-clock nursing or paramedical coverage is not available. A nearby general hospital is the major provider of needed medical care. The simple day room is used for triage, physical examinations, dressing wounds, physical therapy, sobering up, short-term observation, and simple minor surgical procedures. During the day, a nurse or corpsman ideally is immediately available, either on the premises or on short call, and is available by telephone at night.

In minimum-security state and federal correctional institutions, transportation and accessibility are not great problems. Public facilities provide most of the medical care so that health is not, strictly speaking, a prison problem.

Probably the most common inpatient medical facility in jails and prisons is the infirmary. The prison infirmary is a medical facility more like a college infirmary than a simple day room, but less than a general hospital. Most institutions with fewer than 500 inmates have an infirmary or sick bay rather than a general hospital. Such an infirmary requires the presence of a medically trained person every day and night as long as there are patients in the infirmary. Even when the infirmary beds are empty, the accepted standards call for a medically trained professional to be on call at all times. Although those requirements seem obvious, they are in many cases not observed, and no money or personnel is available. Infirmaries are suited for the treatment of most acute and chronic infections, recovery from surgical procedures, minor overdose or withdrawal symptoms, observation following injury, recovery from fractures, isolation, recovery from most acute diseases, and some forms of diagnostic study.

Prison administrators are reluctant to send sick inmates to hospitals outside the prison, for obvious reasons. The requirements of security demand that extra personnel be assigned to drive the inmate to the outside hospital, to guard him while there, and to monitor all his activities and visitors. Guards do not like this work. Administrators do not like the expense. As a result, many larger prisons, housing 300 to 3,000 inmates, have a hospital with broader, but still limited, capabilities.

Only a large institution, housing 3,000 to 5,000 inmates, can support a large, fully equipped hospital. A modern hospital must have readily available staff anesthesiologists, pulmonary and resuscitation experts, a blood bank, a full-time medical records librarian, sophisticated laboratory support services and, in general, a level of complexity well beyond the ability of any Department of Correction smaller than the federal government to operate.

For correctional authorities, the prison hospital may offer several nonmedical possibilities. For instance, the sanctuary of the hospital, with its locked wards, offers the possibility of enforced segregation or isolation. A trip to the hospital is therefore a way of breaking up disruptive cliques. An enforced stay in the hospital may be used as punishment of unruly prisoners. Just as likely, a chance to stay in the clean, safe, well-ventilated hospital may also be a reward offered by correctional staff for good behavior or favors done.

For the prisoner, the hospital or infirmary may be the center for trafficking in alcohol or drugs. Nurses, physicians, consultants, laboratory technologists, and many other people from the outside world come and go through the rooms of the hospital and infirmary. Opportunities abound for unsupervised communication by inmates with the outside world. The hospital also maintains a store of essential items for the drug trade: chemicals for preparing the drugs, the drugs themselves, and the needles and syringes for intravenous use.

Finally, the hospital is a geographically separate part of the prison. The strict rules governing the rest of the prison may be somewhat relaxed in the more human atmosphere of the prison hospital. This relaxation may be exploited by the inmate, however, as when powerful groups of inmates seize control of the clinic and rule it as their private domain.

With all the possibilities for use and abuse and all the secondary benefits derived by inmates, the health care team, and the prison administrators, it comes as little surprise that prison hospitals and infirmaries are frequently the source of controversy. Correctional authorities ask, "Is this trip to the infirmary necessary?" Providers of medical care say, "Let's get this sick inmate to the best care we can find, in or out of the prison." Custody says, "Wait, there are security details and costs to consider." And the outside hospital says, "Wait, we don't want the inmate, the security guards, or the risk."

TREATING EMERGENCIES

Emergencies are a commonplace occurrence in jails and prisons. Jails and prisons are full-time residential units. People may come in with smoldering medical problems or they may develop severe medical problems while behind bars. Prisons are also work units. In any industrial setting, accidents are a regular occurrence. In the prison industrial setting, they are even more likely because of poor equipment, inadequate design of the workplace, inattention to the work task, or sheer malice on the part of fellow workers or guards. Fights, often with dire consequences, are an ever-present possibility in the workplaces of the prison as well as in the recreational and living areas. Yet, despite the relative frequency of accidents in jails and prisons, these institutions are often ill equipped to deal with medical emergencies.

The smaller institutions, where inmates are held for relatively short times or where few inmates are held at any one time, may not need a separate emergency facility. Because the demand for emergency services is so low, it may simply not be economically feasible to maintain a well-equippped and well-staffed emergency room. Unfortunately, when an emergency occurs, regardless of how infrequently, the full range of emergency services must be available. This dilemma is not well resolved by most small jails except by individual negotiation and ingenuity, sometimes at the expense of the rules for maintaining security.

Even in the larger jails, institutions that have an emergency room, the special considerations of security in the design of prisons often puts the emergency room far from the site of most accidents and injuries. The emergency room is not conveniently located, is too small, and, most important, often does not afford easy access for ambulances should the victim need quick transportation to a more fully equipped hospital.

Equipping an acceptable emergency room is not cheap. The basic equipment includes an electrocardiograph and defibrillator; but often even in institutions that have this necessary equipment in the event of cardiac emergencies, there is no one with the experience and training to use it. The other emergency equipment is also expensive: catheters, naso-gastric tubes, intravenous infusion equipment, serum albumin, dry plasma, equipment for drawing blood, microscope and slides, bacteriologic stains, and equipment for cross-matching blood.

The staff running the emergency room have a hard time keeping equipment up to date and, in fact, have a hard time simply keeping the equipment. Much of it is stolen if it is not kept under lock and key. Once again, the familiar paradox of prison medicine:

emergency equipment must be kept available for immediate use, but if the equipment is kept in the open, ready for use, it is likely to be stolen. If it is kept locked up, either the key is lost or the equipment has mysteriously vanished from its locked area.

OUTSIDE HEALTH CARE FACILITIES

The potential for trouble is always great when prisoners who are too ill or too badly injured to be treated in the prison facility are transferred to an outside hospital. Often no contract exists between the prison and the hospital so that arrangements are made on short notice by administrative personnel. This typically hectic and ad hoc method compounds the medical disaster.

Most large city hospitals have a section permanently staffed by personnel trained in security and accustomed to handling sick and injured prisoners. A maximum-security ward in a local hospital is one arrangement which, although expensive, is highly effective. A locked ward in a general hospital is usually escape-proof. Despite the popularity of this system in the past, there is now a tendency for hospitals to move away from such strict segregation of prison inmates toward keeping inmates on the general ward, but with heavy guard. When a prisoner is transferred to an outside hospital, security is provided by the prison security force, not by the hospital. Preventing escape should not become the hospital's responsibility.

Treating prisoners on the general ward has advantages and disadvantages. Guarding a single patient around the clock is expensive for the corrections department. It is also undesirable from the point of view of the hospital administration to have armed guards around the clock to prevent escapes.

The essence of emergency care is rapid identification of a problem and transfer of the patient to a definitive treatment center. In prison, the time between determining that an inmate should be taken to an emergency general hospital for such conditions as deep stab wound, heart attack, or pulmonary embolus and the time that the patient is on the road to the local hospital is rarely less than half an hour. Guards must be found to take the sick patient to the hospital, someone must summon an ambulance, a guard must inspect the empty ambulance and review the guards who will be taking the sick prisoner to the hospital. Medical staff must assemble the relevant records and get the patient into the ambulance. Then the loaded ambulance must pass through the several security checks dictated by prudence and mandated by law.

Still escapes and attempted escapes are often associated with medical transfers. Transportation officers must be alert to the possibility that the trip to the hospital may give the prisoner, sick as he might be, the chance to escape. At the same time, these same officers must not forget that they are transporting an extremely sick person, too, and must be prepared to administer emergency first aid if the patient's condition worsens en route.

The equipment used to transport sick inmates from the prison to the local hospital often leaves a great deal to be desired. In some instances, prisons use commercially licensed ambulances, which are well-equipped and well-maintained emergency vehicles. When their staffing is equal to the sophistication of the equipment, these ambulances provide excellent and safe transportation, though offering little security. More often, however, the prison system uses its own vans to transport sick prisoners to the hospital. These vans are usually heavily armored but poorly equipped with emergency medical equipment or supplies.

SPECIALIZED HOSPITAL CARE

Special hospitals are available for inmate-patients with special needs. Sexual offenders and emotionally disturbed inmates are sent to special hospitals. Drug-dependent and alcohol-dependent inmates, on the other hand, are almost never sent to hospitals specially designed to treat their conditions. As a result, except for the largest city jails and federal prisons, with a large population of drug-addicted inmates, few programs are available inside the prisons and no programs outside the prisons are utilized. Problems of drug and alcohol dependency are therefore treated by the in-house medical staff along with all the other medical and psychological problems.

Departments of mental health and correction have what often

seem to be reciprocal relationships. When mental hospitals are emptied by the economic measures (cloaked as they are in the garb of humanitarianism) known as deinstitutionalization, prisons fill up. Bassuk, Rubin, and Lauriat (1985) conclude:

> Another expression of the troubled existence of the homeless is their antisocial behavior reflected by their criminal involvement. Approximately 44% of those interviewed reported that they had been in jail. Somewhat more than ⅔ were indicted for minor offenses probably related to alcoholism, such as drunk and disorderly conduct, disturbing the peace, and misdemeanors. However, the remaining one-third ($N = 9$) said they had been incarcerated for dangerous crimes such as armed robbery, assault and battery, and murder. Of those who had been in jail for all offenses, 56% were chronic alcoholics and 22% had major mental illness.

These data come from a census conducted in Boston and Cambridge on 25 February 1983 of a 100-bed shelter. Although it is certainly beyond the scope of the present discussion to analyze the relationship between institutions for the homeless and institutions for the criminal offender, one striking point to come out of the research is that they do, indeed, serve the same population.

Prison is not a therapeutic environment. Yet very few cities, counties, or states in the United States permit correctional authorities much latitude in placing emotionally disturbed people convicted of crimes or in transferring apparently normal convicts who develop severe emotional disturbances while in prison. Various hospital arrangements have been worked out to care for emotionally ill prison inmates. These institutions may be called correctional mental hospitals, hospitals for the criminally insane, or criminal justice units. The different names reflect the different ways correctional and medical authorities think about emotionally disturbed offenders.

Patients are detained at such institutions for indeterminate and long periods. The stay at a correctional mental hospital is usually far longer than a prison sentence. In the stricter jurisdictions, a prisoner is sent to a correctional mental hospital for a specific diagnosis and treatment plan. Once these are determined, a course of action is mapped, but most hospitals and correctional authorities operate more or less arbitrarily. In the Netherlands, the psychotic criminal offender is detained "at the Queen's pleasure," as they say, and can be released from the prison hospital at any time on the recommendation of the medical staff, after an independent board reviews the evidence and agrees on the disposition of the case.

The British instituted an "open door policy" in 1972–1973 by which psychotic offenders could be sent to an ordinary psychiatric hospital having neither the facilities nor staff to maintain security. "A hospital cannot at one and the same time look forward to a therapeutic community and backwards toward the security of a prison," according to the Butler Committee. The group therefore proposed that each hospital region have a unit of 50 to 100 beds for convicted offenders and other mentally abnormal individuals needing treatment under secure conditions. "Dangerous psychopaths and other patients known to be real security risks would still be detained in a special hospital such as Broadmoor, but these new units would relieve prison medical staff of the task of trying to treat mentally abnormal offenders and prisoners who develop mental illness while serving a sentence." (1974, p. 215).

An institution for the care and custody of emotionally disturbed offenders must have the physical characteristics of a prison so that the maximum security required by law can be achieved. At the same time, the institution must be relatively free of antitherapeutic factors so common in prisons—crowding, neglect, solitary confinement, noise, inadequate light or excessive light, poor ventilation, and enforced separation from family and friends.

Probably the most renowned and successful mental health program for criminal offenders is the one at England's Grendon Prison. Security is kept at a low profile, there are few escapes and few lockups, there is relatively little violent behavior, and, it is said, there is little use of tranquilizers for disciplinary reasons. The recidivism rate was at first said to be low. But a study by John Gunn and others (1982) reported a rate of rearrest after release to be 70 percent—the same as in other British prisons.

In part, the good results obtained at Grendon can be ascribed to careful selection of offenders, but it is also true that the program depends on building a strong sense of community among staff and inmates. The 200 male inmates and seventy staff plus seven psychiatrists, four psychologists, and psychiatric social workers and welfare workers all cooperate to create a model program, which is very costly in terms of manpower and money. When one of the authors (Prout) visited Grendon, he sat in on one of the peer-led group therapy sessions and then had an hour alone with a dozen of the inmates, largely sex offenders. The most striking feature was the inmate-enforced discipline, neatness, and orderly conduct. To visiting correctional officials, these were "model" prisoners. Several of them pointed out that this restrained behavior was a condition of being permitted to stay the full one (rarely two) years at Grendon. None of the group felt that his behavior after release would be substantially different as a result of his experience at Grendon. One said, "But now I know how not to get caught."

The alternative to the Grendon program is a locked ward or security unit in a civilian hospital. This method has the advantage of providing care by a staff experienced in treating many types of mental and emotional disorders. It has the further advantage of being removed from the harsher aspects of the correctional institution. Nevertheless, such institutions are not well equipped to deal with the special problems of the criminal inmate, notably violent behavior. Better results are sometimes obtained by keeping the emotionally disturbed inmate in a smaller prison or small prison hospital, where communications are easier and security arrangements can suit the needs of the inmate and the correctional system.

Many states maintain special hospitals or segregated units for inmates convicted of such crimes as rape, sodomy, child abuse, or sexually motivated murder. Treating such offenders is difficult, however, because of the mixture of psychological, drug-induced, and hormonal factors to be sorted out in the diagnosis and management of the patient. Such sexual offenders cannot de facto be identified as high- or low-risk inmates. In fact, much evidence now suggests that sexual offenders cannot be differentiated from any other violent or disturbed inmates. As a practical matter, such inmates (most of whom are male) are segregated for their own protection. Fellow inmates, as the Pinero play *Short Eyes* made painfully clear, resent and loathe sex offenders. Inmates convicted of sexually abusing young children are especially vulnerable to judgment and violent attack by their prison peers. For their own good, therefore, sexual offenders are usually segregated from the rest of the prison population.

SURGERY

The line between emergency procedures and routine surgery is fine and often open to argument. Surgeons and other members of the medical team should be the ones to decide whether a surgical procedure is emergency or elective. Since all but the simplest surgical procedures are performed in large general hospitals outside the prison, often the decision is not made on medical grounds at all but on nonmedical, administrative grounds. Correctional authorities, almost without exception, prefer to have surgery carried out within the prison because of the lower costs, ease of maintaining security, saved resources and personnel, reduced paperwork, and the opportunity to keep track of the inmate-patient's medical progress without possible interference by outside medical personnel.

In general, except for the very few prison hospitals accredited by the Joint Commission (see chapter 7 for a discussion of the accrediting procedures), no surgical procedure should be performed in a prison hospital if it requires general anesthesia or might require an assistant, blood transfusions, blood gas measurements, or skilled postoperative follow-up.

Even in a large, well-equipped prison general hospital, accredited by the Joint Commission, anesthesia is hard to provide on demand. There will not be enough demand for an anesthesiologist to warrant hiring one full-time. The best arrangement is often to contract with a local group of anesthesiologists to provide complete coverage as needed. Unfortunately, however, the services of an anesthesiologist are often underpaid so that recruiting for a prison service is often difficult and needed surgery is delayed.

In view of the growing complexity of surgical procedures and the increasing costs, not to mention the rising standards and threat of suit in the event of untoward outcome, few prison hospitals are willing to make the investment needed to prepare an adequate surgery. Staff, house officer coverage, laboratory facilities, intensive care unit, recovery room, blood bank, and anesthesia are all more readily available and more economically provided by a large general hospital. Only the simple general surgery is left for the prison hospital.

THE LABORATORY

As the practice of medicine has become more "scientific," the medical laboratory has become the most visible index of the quality of medical care. Clinical chemistries testing and other sorts of laboratory tests are now an essential feature of acceptable modern medical practice. Except for the laboratories found in large federal prisons and in the larger state and city prisons—and arrangements like those at Rikers Island in New York under contract with Montefiore Hospital and Dade County in Florida under contract with the University of Miami Medical School—most prison medical systems have inadequate laboratory facilities and insufficient funding to buy outside laboratory services.

In the defensive medicine practiced today, physicians order tests to protect themselves against the possibility of a future malpractice suit should the treatment not go as expected and desired. When the prison medical staff is certain that they will be defended by the correctional authorities and by the prison medical administrators, the number of tests ordered falls remarkably. If the medical team is aware of the proper indications for various medical tests, this restricted use of tests may improve medical care, not impair it.

The minimal laboratory equipment needed for a prison medical facility varies according to the size of the prison and proximity to a good general hospital or commercial testing laboratory. The needs of a day room or small infirmary in a city jail are simple: urine containers, blood-drawing equipment, culture tubes, media for planting cultures from the throat, vagina, anus, or urine, urine test papers, and blood glucose qualitative test paper strips. The medical laboratory of a prison far from a good outside laboratory must also include a centrifuge, a microscope, an incubator, blood counting chamber, stains and slides, equipment for obtaining samples of blood gases, and an automated device for obtaining sophisticated blood chemistries. These are all expensive pieces of equipment.

Anyone can learn to carry out the routine clinical tests. Newer automated instruments do most of the work for the technician so that all one needs to do is prepare the sample for the machine. Nevertheless, many prisons boasting well-equipped prison hospitals and surgeries still lack the personnel to perform the clinical testing. Specimens are still sent out to commercial laboratories or hospitals or, in some instances, to the state or municipal hospital laboratory.

Drug screens or toxic screens are especially important in the prison setting; and even the smallest jail or lockup, where intoxicated inmates are held immediately after being taken from the street, is expected to have the means of testing the newly imprisoned for the presence of drugs and alcohol. Prisoners returning from furloughs and long-term inmates, as well, may be tested for the presence of illicit drugs.

Private agencies, probation departments, and methadone maintenance clinics in every community have or use qualified laboratories to test the urine specimens of their clients. Federal funding for many of these laboratory programs is also available to the prisons. There might be great savings if the prisons developed their own testing laboratories. Unfortunately, communication and coordination are often poor or nonexistent so that prisons use unreliable laboratories and fail to develop their own drug screen or toxic screen programs.

X-ray equipment is also useful for the prison hospital but costly to buy and maintain. The relatively high incidence of peptic ulcer and trauma in prisons as well as the necessity of screening for tuberculosis argue for having X-ray equipment in the larger prison hospitals. Radiologists are the highest paid medical specialists, however, so that obtaining the services of a visiting radiologist is an expensive proposition. Films may be taken in the prison, however, and then referred to the local radiologist for interpretation; but more often the inmate-patient is taken to the radiologist—with all the risks and expenses already outlined whenever an inmate is taken out of the prison.

MEDICAL RECORDS

The medical record is the standard by which all medical care is judged. The record protects the patient and the physician, and yet the most important pages of inmates' medical records have an almost uncanny way of disappearing from the folder.

Confidentiality of the medical record is an important consideration. The inmate-patient's record containing information which might block his early release might be revealed or details of his sexual or drug orientation might become known to the general prison population. Guards or other inmates might want someone's record for blackmail. Orderlies, nurses, or physicians might wish errors of judgment to be camouflaged. Yet, until recently, maintaining the confidentiality of inmates' health records was not considered a high priority, and it became necessary for AMA standards to specify this as one of the most essential features for certification of prison medical facilities.

WHAT DETERMINES THE CHARACTER OF A JAIL?

Prisons vary greatly in size, location, and type of inmates they house. All these factors profoundly affect the medical requirements of the facility and the inmates. Some inmate populations, for instance, the so-called criminally insane, violent sexual offenders, and others whose medical conditions and legal status are closely related, pose special problems for the medical care team in prisons.

There are approximately 3,400 lockups and jails in the United States holding an estimated 225,000 prisoners, most of whom are awaiting arraignment and trial. These people have not been sentenced and are, therefore, usually segregated from the convicted criminals, yet they represent some of the most acute and serious problems for the health care team. Physical or mental illness, drug or alcohol intoxication, withdrawal effects as new inmates are deprived of drugs or alcohol, suicidal depression in the first hours of imprisonment, contagious diseases, and other problems all come to the fore as prisoners are presented to the medical system in the jail or lockup.

For some prisoners, introduction to the jail health regimen is often their introduction to the medical care system in general. Usually medical and psychological problems become apparent in the first screening of the inmate population. Because inmates are not kept in the intake facility for long and may even be lost to the system entirely if they are acquitted or paroled, the likelihood of continued treatment of medical problems discovered in the intake screening is low indeed. In fact, few correctional systems make the effort to treat even serious disorders they discover in the lockup— unless those disorders are immediately life-threatening or likely to involve the correctional system in litigation for neglecting them.

The character of correctional institutions is determined, to a large extent, by the size of the prison or jail. Most municipalities have a lockup no bigger than a few cells. The average daily census of these small, local jails may be very small. Many days, there may be only one person; some days, no one at all. The large, long-term federal and state prisons, on the other hand, may house from 500 to 8,000 prisoners. The median is about 1,000. County prisons fall between the small local lockups and the large state and federal prisons. They generally hold between 100 and 1,000 inmates.

The quality of medical care is frequently determined by the size of the institution. The largest may have the physical and financial resources to provide good care; but the smaller jails and lockups, perhaps lacking the large budgets of the large institutions, nevertheless more consistently offer the best care. The largest correctional institutions are almost always located in the countryside, far from urban centers. As a result, it is often hard to recruit the best medical personnel. Referral centers for the more complex cases are far away from the prison. Because of the sheer size of the large prisons, management problems often overwhelm the system for providing medical attention. Taken all together, the problems of size, personnel, and access to the rest of the supporting medical system severely hamper even the most energetic efforts to provide good medical care.

In contrast, the smaller institutions are often in a position to provide care quickly, efficiently, and with the personal attention that all good medical care requires. Under the best circumstances, the prison physician is an able and mature general practitioner or general surgeon who enjoys good relations with the administrators of the prison and with the local hospital and medical community. We have known many such physicians. They can get things done quickly and humanely without the overwhelming paperwork and formality required by large medical systems.

Larger systems require accountability. Small institutions are still personal enough to get along by word of mouth. Accountability is not a great problem because administrators and health workers know each other, trust each other, and can remember what actions have been taken and what plans have been laid for the future. In larger systems, accountability is a major problem, controlled only by maintaining a well-constructed paper trail. Institutional memory is short; lines of communication get tangled. But the paper trails, unfortunately, often twist and turn beyond recognition.

6
Medical Disorders

Most of the medical conditions that concern the prison medical team are the result of the inmates' personalities, their lifestyles, and their chronic abuse of drugs and alcohol, all of which may not have received adequate medical attention before incarceration. Preexisting or prison-acquired homosexual behavior also may have medical consequences. Because inmates are young, however, the immediately obvious physical effects of individual predisposition to disease, self-abuse, and medical neglect are often relatively minor. Long-term health effects of preincarceration lifestyle become especially important for inmates serving relatively long prison sentences. The cumulative psychological traumas of incarceration and the long-term physical effects of earlier behaviors may eventually pose serious health problems. In these cases, the state or federal correctional departments find themselves paying for the treatment of medical conditions whose roots are in the past, long before imprisonment.

Although prisoners may have had little experience with good medical care before imprisonment, they quickly come to expect good care when they enter the correctional system. Demands on the prison health care system may therefore seem to imply a pressing need when, in fact, the demands may be the result of many nonmedical factors. The number of visits to the infirmary may reflect any of the many secondary gains prison inmates can get from attending sick call—opportunities to complain and get sympathetic attention, requests for medicine and particularly sedative and narcotic drugs, special diets to relieve the tedium of

179

routine prison fare, time off from work details, or, in some instances, transfers to other institutions for health reasons.

There have been few reliable evaluations of the medical status of prisoners. For example, comparing the number of articles on selected medical topics listed in *Index Medicus*, a comprehensive listing of current medical research reports, and the number of articles related to prisoners is revealing (table 1). There are very few studies of prison health.

Several possible explanations for the scanty literature on prison health are: (1) It is extremely hard to recruit physicians to work in correctional institutions. The working conditions in such institutions remain appalling despite significant progress in remedying the situation in recent years, so few physicians seek prison work. (2) There is rarely enough money for adequate medical records systems, and maintaining the confidentiality of these records is always a problem. The inmate-patient is often well aware of the common breaches of security and is therefore reluctant to divulge sensitive information. (3) There is little free give and take of information between the physician and patient. The inmate is likely to regard the physician as an adversary rather than an ally. When the inmate does regard the physician as an ally, it is often as a potential dupe to allow the inmate special privileges on the basis of medical need. Finally, (4) few prison physicians are trained in methods of medical research. Of those who are, few are motivated strongly enough or remain in the system long enough to make careful observations and report them in the scientific literature.

Research workers are usually not welcomed by prison inmates; nor are they welcomed by administrators or guards. Prison inmates and guards often share an unusual complicity in keeping information from outside investigators. Inmates withhold information, fearing that incriminating information might be discovered in their medical records. Guards, for a variety of reasons, are likewise reluctant to offer outsiders a glimpse of health conditions within their jails and prisons. We can only speculate on the reasons for this reticence. Perhaps they are simply defensive and fearful when asked, expecting outsiders to be less than sympa-

TABLE 1.   *Number of Studies in the Current Medical Literature*
on Selected Illnesses in Jails and Prisons

	Total No. of Reports	Reports on Prisoners' Health
All medical literature	400,000–500,000	Fewer than 150
Brain disorders	63,050	0
Hypertension	34,750	2
Diabetes	18,277	1
Gastrointestinal illness	17,465	6
Hepatitis	25,849	31
Suicide	12,999	40
Tuberculosis	11,568	21
AIDS	6,240	12
Cirrhosis	6,013	1
Peptic ulcer	4,853	0
Syphilis	2,256	3

Source: Compiled by the authors.
Note: Approximately one million prisoners are admitted each year.

thetic listeners to their side of the story. Perhaps they want, more than anything, to protect the status quo and would rather not give encouragement to any forces of change. Regardless of the reasons, the fact remains that accurate and precise information about health conditions inside jails and prisons is extremely difficult to come by.

In addition, medical records are often lost or incomplete. Clerical personnel are usually overworked and simply cannot keep up with the necessary paperwork. Where possible, medical and clerical staff will take shortcuts in the tedious process of record keeping just to keep pace with the flow of records to be written and filed. Records may also be stolen for the purposes of blackmail or self-protection. Or, most likely, records are simply not filled out by the overworked and undermotivated staff.

Medical investigators have only sketchy information with which to compare inmates' health before, during, and after prison. Most prisoners have found their medical services (if at all) outside the conventional medical system. As a result, most inmates have left no medical records behind when they crossed from civilian life to prison life. Even when medical records are maintained, they may be systematically skewed. In one prison survey, for instance, all emergencies at the prison were sent out to a local emergency ward and, consequently, were not counted in the summary of prisoners' medical conditions. According to the medical records, that facility had very few medical emergencies. In another prison survey, drug- or alcohol-related diseases were not included in the tabulation of medical disorders treated. In yet another, inmates in solitary confinement were not included with other prisoners in regular medical reports. Finally, mental illness statistics may be distorted by pretrial diversion of mentally ill people or by presentence management of mentally ill convicts, both practices vary from place to place.

We do have enough anecdotal clinical information, however, to be able to say that there are some distinct and highly significant differences between the general population and the prison population, particularly those inmates who have been in prison several times. It is not immediately clear whether these differences are the result of imprisonment or are conditions that existed prior to imprisonment. We can only assert that prison medicine is different from other branches of medicine and that the health of prisoners has several peculiar features that cry out for further research.

Prison produces no unique diseases. No disease processes seen in prison are not also seen outside. Some medical, surgical, psychological, or dental problems may be seen more frequently in prisons, some may be more severe because of neglect both before and during incarceration, and some may be presented differently by the prison inmate. However, with only a few notable exceptions to be discussed below, the problems of medical management within prisons are primarily those of circumstance and not biology. Surveys of health problems among prison populations almost invariably show the following:

- The incidence of serious diseases is lower than expected.
- Psychosomatic complaints are very common.

- Liver disease is common.
- Peptic ulcer and ulcerlike symptoms are common.
- The incidence of contagious disease, with the possible exception of tuberculosis, is low, although the incidence of tuberculosis in jails and prisons may be no different from that in a comparable population outside prison.
- The medical complications of drug abuse are widespread and severe.
- Alcohol dependence is a major problem and has been underreported in the past.
- Psychological and psychiatric problems are common among prison inmates and may be made worse (although, paradoxically, sometimes better as well) by imprisonment.
- The incidence of hypertension is significantly lower among long-term prison inmates than among the general population.

We are concerned in this chapter primarily with diseases as they relate to imprisonment (realizing that they are found outside prisons as well) and with the peculiar features of treating diseases when treatment is limited by the constraints of security. There is no substitute for taking a close look at concrete details of the problem in trying to formulate solutions to the problem. We recognize that the expert, who must deal daily with these problems, is more interested in a practical listing of medical disorders in jails and prisons. We also recognize that even the general reader, who has come this far in attempting to understand the combination of care and punishment in prison medical practice, wants to understand the medical problems that prison medical staffs must treat. It is too easy to offer ideal solutions to problems presented in the abstract. Too often, however, these ideal solutions suffer from defects, once identified by H. L. Mencken, of most wishful thinking presented in the guise of recommendations: they are simple and elegant but wrong.

SEX IN PRISON

Nowhere does the tension between care and punishment produce more confusion and polarization of liberal and conservative approaches to prison health care than in the management of sexual mores, behavior, and actions of prison inmates. We know very little about sexual behavior in general, in or out of prison, and the hydraulic model of sex seems to be the only one that can find widespread acceptance. According to this overly simple model, sexual pressure builds (how and what this "pressure" might be is still not clear) and seeks an outlet. In prison, the heterosexual outlets are blocked. We intend no moral judgment of heterosexual behavior versus homosexual behavior. Our only interest here is in the health factors associated with sexual practices in prisons.

In those Latin countries where conjugal visits are an accepted practice, it is said that unrest and psychological problems associated with homosexual behavior are less frequent. In prison, homosexual liaisons are associated with jealousy, hostility, and power struggles. This is true of both men's and women's homosexual relationships in prison. On the other hand, the tendencies toward depression, anger, and poor self-image—almost universal among prison inmates—are apparently reduced risks for inmates who have sexual contact. Heterosexual conjugal visits are permitted in only twenty-one state prisons in four different states—California, Mississippi, New York, and South Carolina. In California, limited conjugal visits have also been permitted to homosexual partners.

The medical community is as confused as the rest of society about homosexuality and particularly homosexual behavior in prison. The American Psychiatric Association, for example, classified homosexuality as a disease in the *Diagnostic and Statistical Manual of Mental Disorders* second edition (*DSM*-II) but, in the *DSM*-III, removed "uncomplicated homosexuality" from the list of mental and emotional diseases. An editorial in the *Southern Medical Journal* (1984, pp. 149–50) urged, "Health care providers in this age of unbridled enthusiasm for preventative [*sic*] medicine would do well to seek reversal treatment of homosexual patients just as vigorously as they would for alcoholics or heavy cigarette smokers, for what may not be treated might well be avoided." For the writer of this editorial, homosexuality is a dirty and unhealthy habit. When like-minded physicians are the principal care givers to homosexual prison inmates, the lines between care and punishment become unclear indeed.

Probably the most lurid feature of prison life is the possibility of forced homosexual rape of the newly imprisoned. Despite common belief to the contrary, the perpetrators of such homosexual rapes are usually not established homosexuals but are rather aggressive heterosexuals and bisexuals. A 1978 report by the Federal Bureau of Prisons stated that although homosexuals are frequently the victims, the vast majority of rapes and assaults are committed by persons who are not homosexuals. The assaulters treat the victims "like females." Their targets are young, good-looking heterosexuals and known homosexuals. Nine percent of heterosexual men studied in a medium-security prison in California reported that they had been sexually assaulted. Forty-one percent of the homosexual men had been assaulted. As for the occurrence of homosexual acts in the same prison, 65 percent of the inmates admitted to homosexual activity while there (Wooden and Parker, 1982).

When sex is forced on an unwilling inmate, it is very difficult to find witnesses who are willing to testify, so offenders already behind bars are seldom prosecuted for their further assaults. Dr. Carmen T. Ciatteo, a psychiatrist at the Illinois Department of Corrections, pointed out in his remarks at the National Conference on Correctional Health Care held in Chicago in 1981, "The inmates are afraid to testify. They are afraid their wives are liable to find out whether they were the perpetrators or the victims." It is also possible that in some instances the prison authorities have no great stake in terminating this sort of homosexual behavior because curtailing it might trigger further unrest or violence.

For most of the victims of forcible rape, whether heterosexual or homosexual, the psychological trauma is severe and long-lasting. Given the many indignities of prison life, the physical and psychological effects of homosexual rape can be devastating. The medical team unfortunately can do little to protect and offer help for such victims. As in so many of the conditions we will discuss in this chapter on medical problems in prison, were are grudgingly led to the conclusion that we know too little. Much more research is needed, instead of what now happens: the topic is swept aside or hidden by a conspiracy of silence.

By the same token, it is not clear what the effects of even the most enlightened action might be. An elaborate scheme was set up in California to classify inmates and protect high-risk new inmates from assault. The remedial action, however, was to take the high-risk new inmates identified by the classification system and put them in strict security. This amounted to confining the potential *victims* in maximum isolation, as they were told, "for their own good." Practices like these bring us to question the difference between care and punishment.

AIDS

"In fighting crime, we have become involved in an explosive public health problem," to quote Mario Merola, district attorney for the Borough of the Bronx, New York City. Drug addicts are being incarcerated in an effort to control the epidemic of drug addiction in the United States. Once in jail, their uncontrolled drug habits and, perhaps, homosexual behaviors pose a constant threat of spreading AIDS among the prison population. "Pretty soon, there will not be any debate in this city about overcrowded prisons. AIDS will take care of that" (*New York Times*, 5 March 1987). Of the approximately 50,000 inmates at Rikers Island in 1986, for instance, an estimated 12,000 probably carried the AIDS virus. AIDS is now the leading cause of death in New York State prisons, rising from 3 deaths in 1982 to 124 in 1986.

The transmission of AIDS in correctional facilities needs more study. In jurisdictions with large numbers of AIDS cases, almost all cases (95 percent of the cases in New York, for example) can be traced to intravenous drug abuse combined with homosexual sexual practices.

AIDS is an apparently new contagious disease of multiple causes whose precise mechanisms are still to be clarified. The likelihood of contracting AIDS is related, at least in part, to lifestyle. Intravenous drug abuse and homosexuality are two particularly powerful risk factors for AIDS, and both intravenous drug abuse and homosexuality are likely components of the inmate's lifestyle out of prison as well as in. The incidence of the disease is therefore much higher among prison inmates than among the general population.

The disease is also now seen with increasing frequency in women. Mortality for men and women alike is exceptionally high, approaching 100 percent. Death occurs within two years in well over half the cases. Because there is no cure at this time, the emotional impact of the disease is enormous, both inside and outside the walls.

AIDS was first recognized about 1981. Within two years, more than half the reported cases were identified in prisons in the New York City area. The groups then at greatest risk were homosexuals and intravenous drug abusers. It became clear that Haitians and the sexual partners of known AIDS cases were also at increased risk. According to a report issued by the National Institute of Justice (NIJ) of the U.S. Department of Justice and the American Correctional Association (ACA) (Hammett, 1986), a total of 766 definite cases of AIDS were identified in U.S. jails and prisons by January 1986. The NIJ and ACA gathered information on the incidence of AIDS in the fifty state correctional institutions, thirty-seven large city and county jails, and the federal prisons by questionnaires. The response from the administrators of these correctional systems was almost perfect; all the state systems replied, as did thirty-three of the thirty-seven city and county systems and the Federal Bureau of Prisons. Twenty-four state prison systems and the Federal Bureau of Prisons accounted for 455 of the AIDS cases; twenty large city and county jails reported 311 cases. These numbers are getting larger with every passing month.

This large population of AIDS victims in U.S. jails and prisons poses a major problem. Approximately one-third of the cases were released from custody. But 23 percent of the reported cases remained in custody and 42 percent of the reported patients had died while in custody.

One curious aspect of AIDS is the sharply limited geographic distribution of the disease. Figures published by the National Centers for Disease Control show that 80 percent of the state and federal correctional systems accounted for only 5 percent of the AIDS cases, while 4 percent of the system contributed 72 percent of the cases. The picture is the same for city and county systems: almost 70 percent of the systems contributed only 5 percent of the cases and 6 percent of the systems contributed 77 percent of the cases. The overwhelming majority of AIDS cases in jails and prisons occur in the Middle Atlantic States. Almost 76 percent of the cases in state systems and almost 72 percent of cases in city and county systems occurred in New York, New Jersey, and Pennsylvania. The next highest incidence rates are far lower than this (11.3 percent in state systems of the South Atlantic states and 16.7 percent in city and county systems of the Pacific states).

AIDS is suspected if an inmate's behavioral patterns put him in a high-risk group and if he shows a history of fatigue and of multiple infections (especially by unusual infecting agents), enlargement of the lymph nodes, and the presence of a previously rare skin cancer known as Kaposi's sarcoma. The most common symptom between the episodes of the various infections is fatigue.

A virus implicated in certain types of human leukemia, the human immunodeficiency virus (HIV), appears to be the first but not the only precipitating cause of AIDS. To make the diagnosis, a logical method would be to screen the inmates by taking the history of intravenous drug use, homosexual behavior, and frequent infections, and then to look for enlarged lymph nodes. Beyond that, the expensive and not entirely accurate test for the antibody to the HIV virus is rarely done as a routine entry screening or even recommended unless, on the basis of these other findings, there is a very strong suspicion of AIDS.

As a result of the difficulties in screening, only six state prisons and seven of the responding city or county jail systems screen (or plan to screen) all new inmates or all present inmates. In most of the other institutions, diagnostic testing for AIDS is reserved for cases in which there is a strong likelihood, on the basis of the physical examination, that the patient is suffering from AIDS. On the other hand, regardless of the difficulties of making an early and positive diagnosis of AIDS, it is desirable to identify and remove cases of AIDS from the general prison population. The problem with removing suspected AIDS cases, however, is that even suspicion of AIDS engenders irrational fear. A false positive test result could be more damaging than a false negative. When the diagnosis of AIDS is known to the patient and other inmates, the problems become worse. The patient fears for his life. He is also rejected and isolated by the other inmates, and fearing contagion, other inmates might even kill the AIDS patient.

Caring for the AIDS patient in the correctional setting requires making fine distinctions between care and punishment, between protecting the civil rights of the inmate with AIDS and protecting the civil rights of the rest of the prison population as well as the civil rights of the broader society. The best way to manage the situation is by strictly isolating the AIDS patient from the other inmates. This isolation is needed to minimize panic more than to prevent secondary cases of the disease. But the need for isolation presents a severe security problem, especially because correctional personnel are often unwilling to care for inmates with AIDS. Isolation also presents psychological stresses of its own.

Limiting visitors and controlling contracts within the prison involves possible infringement of an inmate's rights. The family of at least one inmate (a case in New York) sued successfully for the right to continue visiting an inmate with AIDS. Tracing contacts within the prison, if done aggressively, is not only difficult and expensive, but also involves possible breaches of security and civil rights. Worse still, there is no assurance that the information gathered by such a process would be accurate.

To complicate further the work of the health care team, the disease must be reported by a method designed to preserve confidentiality; but there is very little reason to believe that, in prisons, such medical confidentiality can always be maintained. It is therefore not surprising that many people have a vested interest in not finding new AIDS cases in prisons.

Education is an important part of the effort to deal with AIDS. Staff and inmates are easily frightened by the possibility of an AIDS epidemic in the correctional facility. As a result, almost all of the institutions surveyed by the CDC reported that they had or were developing education on AIDS to staff and inmates. Four-fifths of the institutions already provide some form of education. In these institutions, it is reported that education helped prevent threatened job actions by correctional staff unions and relieved the growing hysteria among the inmates.

Treatment for AIDS is at present experimental and possibly dangerous. Current thinking holds that prisoners should not be used as experimental subjects. The cry of exploiting prison inmates as "human guinea pigs" has essentially stopped human research in prisons. Yet the desperate AIDS victim, in prison or out, will try any treatment that holds even a slight promise of success. The care of a prisoner with AIDS tests the medical profession's ancient ethics and principles of professional conduct to the utmost as it involves giving expensive, difficult, and in the end, fruitless medical care to those rejected and, indeed, hated by the general public. The caregivers must further restrict the few rights and freedoms of the prisoner. This team, charged by law with carrying out this duty, is not highly regarded either by the inmate patients or by the public; yet they are expected to carry out tasks that involve considerable medical knowledge and precision.

Prison officials in many places are attempting to prevent the spread of AIDS within their institutions by dispensing condoms. "The position that I'm taking is not a moral decision," said Richard C. Turner, superintendent of the Northwest State Regional Facility in St. Albans, Vermont. "It's a practical one. It's a disease that obviously can spread, and if there's anything we can do to stop it, then we will" (*Boston Globe*, 4 March 1987). Turner is a pragmatist. The disciplinarian takes a different view. Anthony Travisono, executive director of the American Correctional Association, has criticized programs to distribute condoms among prison inmates: "If proper supervision is maintained," according to Travisono, "there would be no need to distribute contraceptives because there would be no homosexual activity." Perhaps the most realistic comment on providing condoms to inmates was utterd by Eli Adorno, an inmate at Rikers Island, who thought the idea was "totally crazy. Do you think someone who is about to rape you is going to stop and think about a condom? No way."

Each of these views is partially correct. Dealing with a medical problem like AIDS in a prison setting is not a moral issue. It is a medical one. Yet distributing condoms to inmates looks like pampering them when, in the public mind, they should be punished. So-called permissiveness on the part of liberal administrators in regard to the sexual orientation or behavior of staff or inmates is often seized upon by politicians and other public figures as ground for attack. Tightening supervision might be effective if guards could watch the inmates twenty-four hours a day. (which, of course, is impossible). In any event, the added expense and repressive environment within the prison might make such constant surveillance a greater liability than the risk of AIDS. Finally, there is the comment of the inmate: he would be right if most homosexual encounters in jail were forcible rape.

Sexually Transmitted Disease

Sexually transmitted diseases are more common among prisoners than on the street, largely because of the homosexual spread of gonorrhea and secondary (late) syphilis. Estimates of the incidence of venereal disease vary widely from a high of 11.8 percent in the Wisconsin prison system to a low of 2.6 percent in New York City. Among female inmates, pregnancy and venereal disease are common, even among the youngest women prisoners.

The transmission of infection by anal-oral intercourse leads not only to an increased frequency of viral hepatitis among the male homosexual population, but homosexual partners may also spread amebiasis or infections of the enteric bacillary groups (for instance, salmonellosis, shigellosis, and even typhoid fever).

Despite the greater incidence of venereal disease in prisons and jails and despite the relative ease of diagnosing venereal disease, case finding is extremely difficult. The inmate often tries to conceal the clinically relevant facts, fearing revenge on the part of the other inmates or correctional officials having access to the inmate's medical records. Inmates are also reluctant to identify others with whom they have had sexual contact. As a result, getting the necessary clinical information depends to a large extent on the reputation of the medical team for preserving strict confidentiality of such sensitive information. For women inmates there are other considerations. They often resist examinations, especially pelvic examinations. Allegations of forced vaginal and rectal examinations of new female inmates are common. Such examinations are against the law, in fact, and sometimes require legal advice before they can be conducted.

Diagnosis of venereal disease can be complicated by several factors. Vaginitis and cervicitis can be caused by many things; gonorrhea is only one of them. In addition, penile or vaginal lesions may be caused by trauma and may not be the chancres associated with syphilis. Young drug abusers, particularly heroin addicts, may have false positive serological tests for syphilis 20 to 30 percent of the time.

Careful examination and laboratory testing of the newly incarcerated for venereal disease are essential for accurate diagnosis. Testing in jails is often a waste of energy, however, because the inmate is often released or transferred within a few days, before the laboratory has had a chance to incubate the cultures and report the results.

The Health Issues of Women in Prison

Some medical concerns are unique to women. A common cause for alarm among newly imprisoned women, for example, is that their menstrual periods become scantier or cease altogether. This suppression of menstruation often follows excessive stress or deprivation. Although it is frightening, and many female inmates wonder if they are still normal women, they are relieved to learn that menstruation will return.

Many young women enter prison already pregnant. Others become pregnant while in prison, especially when there are liberal furlough programs. For those returning from furlough or parole, a gynecological examination and, if requested, a "morning after" pill are indicated medically. Again rules, laws, and attitudes lead to great inconsistency from one state to another, from one prison to another. For administrative and legal, as well as medical, purposes, obviously the earliest possible identification of a pregnant prisoner is desirable; but would we advocate compulsory pregnancy tests? Is this a violation of the inmate's civil rights? Contraception is not generally available to female prisoners on request in mixed-sex prisons and before furlough and parole, and yet, inmates and correctional authorities have everything to gain by preventing unwanted pregnancy.

For the same reasons one might expect abortion for pregnant women prisoners to be carried out on the same terms as for free women in the community. However, in some jurisdictions, it is illegal to pay for abortions out of public tax money and prisoners are specifically denied funds for therapeutic abortions. In any case, the pregnant inmate requires support and counseling as she decides whether she wishes to continue or abort her pregnancy.

It is well known that for better survival rates for both mother and baby, prenatal care should begin as soon as pregnancy is verified. Except in the rarest of instances, pregnant women now deliver in hospitals outside the prison walls, although older women's prisons had their own delivery services. Most women prisoners give up their babies for adoption. Whether this is done or not, the importance to the mother and baby of the bonding process in the early weeks of life and simple humanity would dictate a period of some weeks on furlough before or just after delivery. Again, issues of security, complaints of pampering inmates, and the desire for clear punishment obscure the issues of providing proper medical care.

The medical complications of pregnancy in prison reflect the backgrounds of the inmates. The more serious problems of pregnant inmates, medically speaking, occur among those who have been heavy users of heroin. Factors that are well known as detrimental to a successful, healthy pregnancy include malnutrition, excessive use of alcohol and drugs, and a high rate of infections past and present of the female reproductive tract. These features are widely represented among the group of long-term women prisoners. Since there are no heroin maintenance programs in the United States and almost no in-prison methadone maintenance programs, the question of continuing heroin in the addicted pregnant inmate is academic.

The pregnant inmate is withdrawn from all narcotics at the earliest possible time. Managing the withdrawal reactions of any addict is a difficult process. Pregnancy greatly complicates the problems. Moreover, many women are jailed shortly before going into labor when they have not been withdrawn from heroin or cocaine. They give birth to addicted babies who are generally small, sickly, and suffer a high death rate.

The dangerous syndrome of neonatal withdrawal shortly after delivery is characterized by a hyperactive baby with tremors, vomiting, a shrill cry, sneezing, yawning, hiccoughing, exaggerated reflexes, and respiratory distress. These signs and symptoms are also seen in the newborn babies of women who are jailed shortly before going in to labor when they have been on heavy doses of barbiturates and alcohol.

ALCOHOL AND DRUGS

Alcohol abuse is an increasingly serious problem among young people in the United States. Consequently, even the youngest prisoners are likely to show some of the problems commonly associated with alcohol abuse: alienation, intoxication, withdrawal symptoms, liver disease, and a history of repeated minor and major accidental and inflicted injuries.

The social values and attitudes of the larger society are important in defining substance abuse and in relating substance abuse to so-called criminal behavior. In Britain and in many city and county jails in the United States, alcoholism and its complications account for more than half of all imprisonments. In other areas, where drunkenness is no longer a criminal offense, alcoholism is not found as the reason for imprisonment. Lawmakers and enforcers who are older and more tolerant of alcohol abuse may soften their treatment of alcohol abusers. By the same token, lawmakers and enforcers who are anxious about drug use in the general population may pass and enforce stringent laws to curtail drug abuse. As a result, drug abuse will appear in prison statistics more frequently and will correlate more strongly with arrest patterns than will alcohol abuse.

Between one-half and three-quarters of the inmates in short- and long-term jails and prisons have abused alcohol. Sixty-five percent of crimes in Maryland, the site of one careful study, were alcohol-related. The sale, possession, or abuse of drugs is one of the major causes for arrest in the United States.

The health of prison inmates and the use and abuse of alcohol and drugs are inextricably bound up with each other. The combined effects of alcohol and various drugs may be greater than the effects of either one taken singly. This synergism leads to profound medical and psychiatric problems that must be attended to when intoxicated offenders are first brought into jails and also leads to major ongoing problems for institutions that must house such offenders for long periods of time.

If prisons could be so tightly controlled that no alcohol or illicit drugs could be found within their walls, the medical management of drug and alcohol problems would be fairly simple. Delirium tremens and abstinence syndromes would be the inevitable, but manageable, medical consequences of taking inmates' alcohol and drugs away from them. There is, however, no drug-free or alcohol-free prison or jail in the United States. The few relatively drug-free institutions are usually small, where the superintendent and chief physician agree to enforce a strict policy of limiting prescriptions for narcotics, sedatives, or amphetamines. Guards, likewise, must be supported in their efforts to control the traffic in contraband drugs. Without such tight controls, efforts to treat alcohol and drug abuse in the inmate population are futile.

The terms *dependence, abuse,* and *addiction* are loosely defined and used even more loosely by some medical and correctional authorities. *Substance abuse* is also largely a social definition, defined by the availability of the alcohol or drugs in the drug-using population and by the attitudes of the larger population. Heroin may be cheap and available in some cities and prohibitively expensive or unavailable in others. In Boston, our study of arrest patterns in 1973 showed that young persons arrested and convicted in certain poor black areas of the city were far more likely to be charged with possession and sale of "heavy" narcotics; young persons arrested in the more affluent white suburbs were more likely to be charged with the lesser offense of possession of marijuana. Actual use of drugs in the two communities was found to be identical.

Alcohol

Alcohol is by far the most commonly used mind-altering substance associated with violent antisocial behavior and is the most common addiction in the United States. Where public drunkenness is considered a crime, short-term jail sentences are heavily biased toward alcohol-related crimes. It is an injustice and unsound medical judgment to assume that an inmate's use of alcohol or drugs—even heavy use—necessarily has led to physical dependence. Dependence is variable in degree and has physical, psychological, and environmental factors. To complicate matters further, alcoholism and alcohol addiction are not synonymous terms.

If alcoholism is defined as any use of alcohol that impairs a person's medical, psychological, social, or vocational functioning, then surely a majority of people in prison must be defined as alcoholics. If alcoholism is defined as a physical or psychological dependence on alcohol, withdrawal of the alcohol should lead to withdrawal symptoms. This is not often the case. Many prisoners show no withdrawal symptoms when deprived of the high levels of alcohol to which they had been accustomed.

By definition, all addictive drugs are associated with abstinence syndromes when they are withdrawn. These physiological or psychological changes may come days or weeks after the last drink, snort, toke, or injection. The medical problems of alcohol or drug abuse in prisons are those of identifying and managing intoxication, detoxification, withdrawal, and abstinence syndromes, rehabilitation, and long-term medical complications resulting from chronic abuse of these substances. Intoxication of the newly imprisoned person is a problem for the booking officer and for the guards and medical team who must manage the inmate-patient through the difficult period of withdrawal.

When first imprisoned, even while being held in a police station, lockup, or city jail, an alcohol-dependent prisoner is at the greatest medical risk of his entire term of imprisonment. The prisoner may become comatose. A reckless adolescent, for example, may overdose shortly before arrest and, during the process of arrest and imprisonment, may go into severe respiratory distress. If not properly attended, the prisoner may die of respiratory paralysis. Also if left unattended, some intoxicated prisoners have choked on their own vomit and suffocated.

A careful medical examination could be crucial at intake. The arresting authorities sometimes assume that all the signs and symptoms shown by the prisoner are directly due to simple alcohol intoxication. The experienced drinker develops some tolerance to alcohol, however, so that the usual difficulties in speaking or walking may not be immediately obvious to the arresting officer or the medical staff doing the intake examination. In the younger inmate, simultaneous overdose of drugs and alcohol is the chief hazard.

Because an immediate medical examination is rarely possible, police or jailers must learn to be aware of the obvious signs of intoxication. Intoxication is only identified if the booking officer suspects it and can tell it from other possible diagnoses as insulin reaction, brain injury, or intoxication by other substances. Such officers with little or no formal medical training fortunately often have a generous share of "street smarts."

The effects of withdrawal from drugs and alcohol are partly physiological, partly psychological. *What* is done to and for the inmate-patient and *how* it is done are both extremely important in detoxifying and rehabilitating a drug- or alcohol-dependent patient. The most serious consequence of withdrawal from alcohol is delirium tremens, which has a mortality rate of 15 percent. The pain and suffering, short of mortality, are immeasurable. Delirium tremens generally occurs after a prolonged and unrelieved period of alcohol consumption. Malnutrition and fatigue exacerbate the symptoms. Within hours or days of the latest drink, the patient becomes restless, sweats heavily, and begins characteristic picking and plucking movements of the fingers with increasing excitement. Prompt action, early in the reaction, may prevent the most debilitating aspects of delirium tremens.

Many jails and prisons have alcohol and drug rehabilitation programs, but programs inside the jails are no more successful than those outside and the failure rate of all alcohol treatment programs is alarmingly high. In the civilian population, Alcoholics Anonymous has been the most widely used and most successful method of treating alcoholism. To be successful in the prison setting, however, AA works best when it uses an inmate team able to communicate with the inmate-patient on his own terms. On the outside, AA functions by asking the person to renounce rebellion. For most prisoners, this is an impossible change of attitudes, and a formidable problem in most prison-based AA programs.

Drugs

Any discussion of drugs and drug use by prisoners is certain to be only approximately correct. There are strong regional differences in patterns of use and abuse. These patterns change rapidly, and, for reasons we have already discussed, studies of drug use are less than perfect. Abuse of a single substance is rare. The effects of abusing several substances at the same time are difficult to unravel.

Heroin use is a major problem among adolescents and young adults. At first, heroin abuse was primarily a problem of the larger urban centers, especially cities in the Northeast and West Coast; but it is now a national problem. Since 1975, the drug has been widely available despite rigorous efforts by law enforcement agencies to restrict the supply. Some long-term prison inmates in the United States are veterans who developed the addiction to heroin and other drugs during their tours of duty in Southeast Asia. Cocaine and PCP (angel dust) abuse are approaching heroin as major causes of medical problems on the street and among prison inmates. Hallucinogens, on the other hand, which may be a major problem outside prisons, are not commonly used inside.

Intravenous injection is by far the most common method of administering heroin in prison as well as outside. The majority of medical complications of heroin abuse, therefore, arise from unsterile techniques of intravenous administration as well as from adulteration of the heroin itself. The most important medical problems associated with the abuse of heroin are as follows:

- Hypersensitivity (allergic) reactions: hives, itching, asthma, life-threatening anaphylaxis
- Cardiovascular effects: hypotension (low blood pressure), heart arrhythmias, endocarditis, phlebitis, arteritis
- Dermatologic effects: itching, abcess, scarring, swelling of the needle sites
- Sexual function: decreased sexual drive, decreased fertility, frequent miscarriages, gynecomastia
- Genito-urinary effects: bloody urine, kidney failure
- Liver effects: hepatitis
- Blood effects: anemia, lymphocytosis, hypergammaglobulinemia, enlarged lymph nodes, false positive serological test for syphilis
- Lung effects: pneumonia, septic emboli, pulmonary edema due to pulmonary capillary leakage
- Nervous system effects: acute brain syndrome, mono- and polyneuropathy, changes in brain waves, respiratory arrest, decreased bladder sphincter tone, flushing, sweating

- Eye effects: quinine amblyopia, talc and cornstarch emboli, metastatic endophthalmitis
- Disorders of pregnancy: prematurity, anemia, premature rupture of membranes, toxemia, abnormal presentation

Pure heroin is a bitter, white crystal. As sold on the street, heroin is colored with various dyes, commonly understood to indicate where the heroin is from. This color coding is less than meticulous. Street heroin is also repeatedly cut with adulterants, of which the most common are quinine, lactose, cornstarch, and mannitol. Other less benign adulterants have been found in street heroin: arsenic, bicarbonate of soda, barbiturates, battery acid, butacaine, caffeine, cocaine, cotton fibers, cyanide, resins and gums, magnesium trisilicate, nicotine, parathione, procaine, talc, and even strychnine. The possible presence of these adulterants presents the medical team managing a case of heroin addiction with the exceedingly difficult task of identifying and evaluating the toxicity of the heroin itself and the many possible adulterants taken along with the heroin.

The diagnosis of heroin use is made by history, physical examination, and laboratory findings. Physical examination alone is not sufficient. The history is subject to the constraints of the inmate's need or desire to withhold information, compounded by the fact that the patient may be no longer competent to give reliable answers to questions posed by the health care team. Injection of a narcotic antagonist (usually Narcan) to neutralize the effects of narcotics on the body can abruptly reverse the effects of heroin. This provides a useful way of diagnosing heroin use and if acute withdrawal symptoms appear, then addiction has been demonstrated as well.

The most useful laboratory test for the presence of heroin is urine chromatography. Few prisons and fewer jails have access to this sophisticated equipment, however, and even this method is not without its technical difficulties. For one thing, the test is obviously invalid if the urine being tested is not from the person being examined. Switching occurs frequently, as inmates attempt to protect each other from the legal consequences of heroin use. It is more difficult, however, for inmates to protect each other from the physiological consequences.

Inmates are familiar with and dread the symptoms of abstinence from drugs and alcohol. The signs and symptoms produced by abstinence from heroin mimic other diseases and can mislead the prison health team. Within a few hours, the patient becomes restless and sweats profusely. Breathing is rapid and short, pupils are dilated, nose and eyes are runny. When the patient goes off drugs "cold turkey," symptoms become most severe within three or four days. After a period that may be from ten hours to ten days, the runny eyes and nose persist along with gooseflesh, gastrointestinal disturbances, rapid pulse, and elevated blood pressure. In all, it may take up to thirty weeks for symptoms of drug withdrawal to disappear completely.

There are several standard protocols for detoxifying newly imprisoned narcotics addicts. State and federal laws, as well as regulations of the U.S. Food and Drug Administration, maintain some control over what can be done to and for imprisoned addicts, especially if methadone is to be used. The Departments of Correction and Health Services Administration in New York City developed their standard treatment protocol in December 1971 and have not altered it substantially in the years since. More than 100,000 heroin addicts have now been treated by the programs described in the New York City protocols. Admittedly, this is a cookbook approach to a complex problem, but one of the virtues of a cookbook is that anyone who can follow the instructions can get an acceptable response. Individual judgment does not become an important factor in the outcome. Of course, opportunities to tailor the programs to the needs of individual addicts are also severely limited.

Some drug workers prefer to have the addict take an active role in his treatment program. This includes having the patient set his own dose schedule. Although there is still no proof of the contention, these workers suggest that a flexible treatment program in a drug-free prison environment, can detoxify an inmate-patient in far less time and with far less methadone than used in the New York protocol. Many prison physicians, particularly physicians in the smaller prisons and jails, where they have more personal contact with inmates and greater opportunities for personal control of the medical situation, favor such a shorter and more intense program of methadone. So great is the disenchantment with methadone in many prisons that medical staffs use no methadone at all and seem to have no bad result.

Methadone treatment programs are a good example of how one addiction can lead to another. Methadone hydrochloride is a narcotic analgesic sold under a number of trade names. The goal of methadone treatment of heroin addiction is to transfer dependence from heroin to a legally and medically controlled substance. It was hoped that physicians and law enforcement personnel could minimize the risks to the addict's health and reduce the traffic in illicit drugs in this way.

Methadone maintenance thus became big business. In 1978, perhaps the high point in methadone maintenance programs, approximately 100,000 addicts in New York City were receiving methadone in federally funded programs at a cost of $1,000 per patient per year. This comes to more than $100 million.

Large city jails and lockups have trouble with newly admitted methadone patients, just as they have trouble with newly admitted heroin addicts. First, jail staff must determine that the inmate is, indeed, a patient in a bona fide methadone treatment program. If he is, staff must decide whether to terminate the therapeutic program and move toward immediate detoxification in prison or to transfer the inmate to a methadone maintenance center under secure conditions.

Methadone maintenance has proved to be highly undesirable in the prison setting. Opportunities are too plentiful for abuse of the substance and loss of medical and administrative control of what should be a treatment program. Where heroin is unavailable, methadone is an acceptable substitute so that addicts will traffic in methadone just as they would have dealt in heroin. Methadone maintenance thus substitutes one administrative problem for another.

Alternatives to methadone in the detoxification of opiate-dependent persons have been proposed. Propoxyphene napsylate (Darvon-N) has been used to ease the discomforts of detoxifying, but the problem with this medication, as with methadone and other substitutes for heroin, is that the substitutes themselves may lead to addiction. Other medications, including the antihypertensive drug clonidine as well as a variety of tranquilizers in decreasing doses are also used in some detoxification programs.

Narcotics are not the only drugs of abuse in prisons and among populations likely to find their way into jails and prisons. Barbiturates are in wide use in the general population. Nembutal, Seconal, Amytal, and Tuinal lead to varying degrees of dependence. Outside prisons, use of these drugs is heavy; inside the jails and prisons, traffic in these contraband drugs is intense. Consequently, the admitting officer in a jail must be attentive to the possibility of barbiturate intoxication and the serious withdrawal symptoms upon deprivation of the drug. Unfortunately, the diagnosis is sometimes difficult. A newly arrested prisoner suffering from an overdose of barbiturates may appear drunk or even unconscious and may die of respiratory depression if not treated appropriately in time. The problem of barbiturates is complicated by the fact that they are often prescribed in prison for their depressant properties. They are cheap hypnotics, tranquilizers, and anticonvulsants, popularly known as "downers" in the argot of the drug users.

Phencyclidine (PCP)—otherwise known as angel dust, goon, busy bee, hog, crystal, or superjoint—was originally developed as an animal tranquilizer but has since found its way into illicit human use. PCP is relatively cheap and easy to manufacture. Variants are often accidentally produced in the process. The drug is easy to administer by sniffing or swallowing.

One-third to one-half of all jail inmates have probably used PCP; one-fifth are probably regular users. This wide use of a variable and unpredictable drug greatly complicates the management of drug-intoxicated inmates. The first effects of PCP (and such variants as PHP) are discomfort in the limbs, then changes in mood with sudden, unpredictable highs to violence and even psychotic rages. Users may attack the nearest person without reason or warning. PCP patients may sometimes appear schizophrenic and are therefore mismanaged. Hallucinations are common. Larger doses of PCP can lead to coma and death.

Amphetamines are common on the street and in prison, usually combined with alcohol or barbiturates. Known as speed, a member of this group of drugs gives the sense of euphoria, wakefulness, diminished hunger, and a sense of profound mental and physical strength. The principal substances used are amphetamine (bennies), dextro-amphetamine (dexies), and meta-amphetamine (crystal). In combination with heroin or methadone, amphetamine or cocaine is known as speedball.

Symptoms of amphetamine intoxication include repeated touching and picking at the hands and face, paranoia, intense introspection, repetitive speech and behavior, and hallucinations. These symptoms may last for days or even weeks. Although signs and symptoms are reversible when the drug is withdrawn, recovery may take considerably longer. During the recovery period, the intoxicated inmate-patient must be observed carefully. Such patients easily become agitated, committing violence against property, other prisoners, and themselves.

Cocaine is a major problem in the jails and prisons, although until relatively recently it was too expensive for most prisoners. Substitutes for the more expensive cocaine have been developed that give some of the same effects of euphoria and excitation. These cocaine substitutes may contain local anesthetics, caffeine, ephedrine, yohime, or inert material.

In addition to illicit drugs, several routinely prescribed drugs have become medical problems in jails and prisons when the drugs are no longer under medical control. Propoxyphene (Darvon, Dolene), methaqualone (Quaalude, Sopor), and meperidine (Demerol) have all entered the street and prison market. Pentazocine (Talwin) was touted as an analgesic with few if any addictive properties. Nevertheless, in the disturbances at Walpole Prison in 1972, as many as 250 of the 650 inmates were routinely using Talwin. Ridding the system of the drug—both the correctional system and the inmates' physiological system—evoked violent responses from inmates and significant resistance among the long-term correctional personnel who had developed their own feelings of hopelessness and helplessness about remedying the drug situation.

Liver Disease

One important function of the liver is to remove foreign substances from the blood. The steady barrage of drugs and alcohol, to which most prison and jail inmates have subjected their livers, thus eventually causes serious damage. The varieties of adulterants in injected heroin, previously mentioned, all lodge in the liver. The liver damage from alcohol is made worse by years of inadequate diet, especially a diet deficient in protein. Abstinence from alcohol (along with bed rest and sufficient nutrition) is a cardinal rule in the treatment of such liver diseases as cirrhosis and alcoholic hepatitis; but even this simple treatment is virtually impossible in prison. Drugs and alcohol are readily available, and many inmates are not sufficiently concerned about their own health and welfare to abstain voluntarily. In this setting, there is little the health care team can do.

Hepatitis is a more complex group of diseases and offers more complex problems to the health care team in prison than cirrhosis, which is the scarred end stage of many processes. The hepatitis virus is transmitted by several routes. It is commonly injected by intravenous drug abusers using contaminated equipment or drugs. It is also a common risk among homosexual males because it may be transmitted by penile-anal-oral intercourse. These means of transmission favor the more dangerous, often lethal virus of hepatitis B. Liver function tests in one jail survey we participated in were abnormal in more than 80 percent of the inmates tested.

Between one-third and three-quarters of all heroin addicts show signs of liver disease. Drug abusers are likely to have several different forms of liver disease because of the unsterile materials they use and because of the chemical contaminants they inject along with the drugs. Amphetamines and some other drugs of abuse are toxic to the liver.

Although living conditions are crowded and would appear to encourage the rapid spread of hepatitis, true epidemics of the disease within prisons have not been reported. In one Massachusetts prison, a kitchen worker was found to have an active case of hepatitis; but after an anxious six months of close observation, no cases appeared that could be traced to inmates' exposure to this carrier. Nor was there any detectable increase in the occurrence of hepatitis in the general prison population.

One explanation for this curious fact is that prisoners are probably already immune to the common viruses of hepatitis by the time they enter prisons and this can be confirmed by testing their blood for hepatitis antibodies. The first attack of the usual infectious hepatitis comes younger in members of the lower socioeconomic groups and older in members of the higher socioeconomic groups. Most prisoners are therefore likely to have developed immunity to many strains of hepatitis by the time they become prison inmates.

Routine screening for signs of hepatitis virus or for prior exposure to hepatitis virus and hence immunity to the disease is seldom carried out because of the prohibitive expense of the procedure. In any event, rest and isolation are easily arranged inside the prison and add little to the cost of maintaining and caring for the prison inmate. The problems in treating liver disease in prison are not the problems of medical management, for they are treated in prison as they would be treated anywhere. That is, by rest. The problems of treating liver diseases in prison are the social and political ones of affording prison inmates such long periods of uninterrupted respite from their usual unpleasant routine.

Most hospitals in the United States have difficulty imposing strict isolation on infectious hepatitis patients. The principal risks are in disposing of stool and urine specimens. In addition to these technical problems, there are the human difficulties of isolating the patient. Visitors must wear masks and gowns. In some hospitals, visitors are excluded completely. In the understaffed prison hospital, however, precautions to isolate the infectious hepatitis patient are time-consuming, difficult, and even leave the medical staff open to charges of inflicting cruel and unusual punishment in their attempts to isolate the patient from staff, friends, and loved ones.

PSYCHIATRIC AND NEUROLOGIC DISORDERS

Some organic disorders of the nervous system are seen with particular frequency in prisons: seizure disorders (epilepsy), effects of alcohol abuse (neuritis and Korsakoff syndrome), effects of drug abuse, and the results of trauma. Many of the disorders of the nervous system reveal themselves as so-called soft signs that are neither specific nor provable (for instance, confusion, headache, drowsiness or sleepiness, clumsiness, or thick speech). Distinguishing the true sign from the feigned requires the greatest diagnostic skill and understanding of the constant possibility that the inmate-patient is simply trying to manipulate the physician. As with so many other medical conditions, the inmate and his associates are usually reluctant to give the examiner a true history, so the medical team must base its decisions on probability and suspicion.

Neurologic Disorders

Headache, of course, is one of the most common symptoms in prison as well as out. It is also one of the most difficult clinical signs to evaluate, for headache may be the sign of serious, life-threatening conditions or headache may simply be feigned in order to get drugs, attention, or release from work. Nonetheless, it is a sad fact that severe emotional strains, deprivations, suppressed hostility, and closed confinement—all common features of prison life—can produce functional headache. These headaches may not be life-threatening but they are nevertheless real, debilitating, and worthy of medical attention. Medical diagnosis of headache, therefore, must rest on the most informed clinical guesses. After all, at the very least the steady discomfort of a headache can make the inmate irritable, and an irritable inmate easily becomes a troublesome and dangerous one.

Organic brain syndrome is a loosely defined term taken to mean abnormal behavior, thinking, or feeling that can be associated with abnormal functions of brain tissue. Organic brain syndrome is a term used to refer to a cluster of signs and symptoms seen most often among older alcohol abusers who have had repeated attacks of delirium tremens, among people who have suffered severe injury to the head, and as a result of chronic malnutrition. The term is anathema to neurologists, but it is still useful to forensic psychiatrists and correctional officials.

People with organic brain syndrome function poorly in many areas of life. They have grossly inadequate personal and social skills. After several years, they are often wholly unable to live on their own. Many of them are repeatedly imprisoned for violent and antisocial acts or are put on the back wards of large mental hospitals. Recovery is extremely rare. Treatment is usually limited to custodial care, and the only two institutions equipped to deal with organic brain syndrome patients are the mental hospitals and the prisons. Deinstitutionalization of the mental hospitals thus throws these unfortunate people into the prisons, where detailed neurologic evaluation is rarely possible and seldom carried out.

Seizure disorders—both grand mal epilepsy and other forms of seizures—are an especially difficult cluster of neurological problems to treat in prisons. For one thing, they are represented in the prison population with a higher frequency than in the general population. This has been most carefully studied by John Gunn in England and, to some degree, in the United States.

The causes may include genetic factors, multiple trauma, and such environmental factors as drug abuse, but evidence is lacking to make a conclusive case. Perhaps the higher frequency of seizure disorders observed in the prison population may be explained, in part, by the fear and discrimination the outside population has often shown toward people with seizure disorders. Such time-honored and unjust punishment of the victim may, to some extent, force him into antisocial behaviors. It is also possible that seizure disorder and antisocial behavior are functionally related, but without much needed research, any supposed relationship between the two is mere conjecture.

Several people, since research done by Ervin and others in the 1960s, have tried to find a connection between outbursts of violent rage and temporal lobe epilepsy (now called complex partial seizures). No definitive study has shown conclusively that temporal lobe epilepsy is more frequent in prisons than outside, and it is a difficult diagnosis to confirm. As a result, there is little positive fact to connect the brain disorder with the behavioral disorder.

Nonetheless, there has been considerable support in the past for a simple and direct treatment of temporal lobe epilepsy. Psychosurgery—surgical procedures for disconnecting or removing parts of the brain that control emotions—has been attempted in an effort to reduce outbursts of violent rage. Despite the simplicity and directness of the surgical approach, it was used only briefly and not widely attempted. Controlled studies of the outcome of psychosurgery have now largely discredited it as a useful approach.

More often, neurologic and behavioral problems are treated with drugs. The physician newly introduced to the setting of prison medicine is often surprised at how frequently antiepileptic drugs, anticonvulsants, and sedatives are prescribed. It is easier and cheaper to prescribe a drug than to carry out a complete, definitive neurologic examination.

Psychiatric Problems

"We judge an artist by his highest moments but a criminal by his lowest," said George Bernard Shaw. In fact, many of an inmate's psychiatric problems may be based on reality. Prison life is enough to drive anyone crazy. The boredom, deprivation, isolation, and alienation make even the simplest forms of gratification difficult. For these reasons all but the most passive inmates are deeply angry.

Comparisons of mental illness in the general population and mental illness in the prison population are difficult and often misleading. By definition, convicted criminals have behavior disorders. By virtue of the social context in which they find themselves, prison inmates lead distorted social and personal lives.

Imprisonment is a potent stressor to most people, but it does not affect all people equally. Some people actually seek the protection of prison, where they can have their dependency needs met. Every experienced judge and probation officer has seen instances of people who deliberately break the law in order to be imprisoned. These people function better in prison than in the unstructured world outside and are model prisoners. They rarely develop acute mental problems in prisons because their basic personality structures suit them to prison life.

Treating such prisoners presents a paradox. The immediate risk of exacerbating mental illness in these people is low. At the same time, however, their chances of adapting to life outside the prison are also low. Teaching them to adapt better to outside life may make them less manageable in the context of the prison to

which they are so well adapted. What is the prison p
service to do?

For most people, however, the stresses of imprisonme
legion and may provoke violent reactions. Most prisoners ac
feel

- Separation from family, friends, loved ones
- Loss of freedom regarding space, time, occupation, recreation, companions, and so forth
- Necessary adaptation to new lifestyles and regimentation
- Aggressive and offensive behavior by other inmates
- Threats by guards and inmates
- Homosexual seductions and threats
- Drug withdrawal
- Anxiety about trial and sentencing
- Shame and guilt, which tend to disappear as imprisonment continues

These and other less obvious stressors can precipitate a variety
of reactions. The length of time it takes a newly imprisoned person to adapt to prison life is variable and some prisoners never do
adapt. It is in the lockups and holding jails that we find most
murderous rages, suicidal gestures, schizophrenic episodes, psychotic decompensation, panic states, and profound depressions.

Estimates of how many prisoners have psychiatric problems
will vary with the prevailing view of how much deviant behavior
is a medical rather than a social problem. Although relatively few
long-term prisoners are clearly psychotic, estimates of the proportion of prisoners showing diagnosable psychiatric problems range
from 5 to 80 percent. Deinstitutionalization of once-hospitalized
mental patients accounts for some of the mental illness found in
prisons. As more mental hospitals refuse admittance to patients
with deviant behavior, people who would have been inmates of
hospitals become inmates of prisons. In Massachusetts, the numbers in mental hospitals and in prisons have been nearly reciprocal. As one population is reduced, the other increases.

The medical team needs a classification for mental disorders
quite independent of the needs of the judicial system. Classifying
emotional or mental disturbances among prison inmates depends
on the objectives of the person doing the sorting. For instance,

classifications acceptable to the criminal justice system do not necessarily correspond to current psychiatric classifications. Current psychological theory has moved away from labeling patients (as, for instance, schizophrenic, paranoiac, and so forth) toward describing the dynamics of individual behavior. This newer approach unfortunately requires more time and is impracticable in large prison settings. Like it or not, a simple descriptive label is easier to deal with on medical and legal forms than a short biography.

One excellent device for arriving at psychiatric diagnoses, the *Diagnostic and Statistical Manual of Mental Disorders* (*DSM*-III) contains many decision trees capable of leading trained observers to consensus on a particular diagnosis. Yet the authors of *DSM*-III warn that use of the classification scheme they have devised to determine "legal responsibility, competency, or insanity" is beyond the scope of the classification scheme. No simple guidebook to psychiatric diagnoses, regardless of how carefully constructed, can lead the untrained observer to reliable diagnoses.

The virtue of *DSM*-III is that it undercuts the common faith that such medico-legal labels as insanity are strictly applicable and that the behaviors of the person to whom such a medico-legal label is attached will be predictable. This is rarely the case, for the human being is far too complex to permit such reductionist labels.

We do not know as much as we would like about the psychodynamics or personality structure of prisoners because these are people who have always distrusted medical authority and have had little exposure to good medical and mental health care. They do not voluntarily subject themselves to testing and interviewing. Nor do we know as much as we would like about the cognitive status of prison inmates. There are few precise data available on the frequency of dyslexia and other grave defects of communication in the general prison population. Most students of the matter agree, however, that the incidence of reading, writing, and speaking problems, for whatever reasons, is far greater among prison inmates than among the general population outside prisons. Yet it is not proven that the average prisoner is measurably less intelligent than his nonimprisoned peers.

Most prison inmates suffer from those ill-defined conditions known as character disorders, psychopathic personality disorders, or sociopathic personality disorders. The official term used by the *DSM*-III is antisocial personality disorder. Inmates are also likely at the same time to have drug and alcohol problems as well as affective disorders (manic-depressive illness, depression, or anxiety).

An adult career of antisocial behavior may be predicted, according to several studies of juvenile delinquents by Eleanor and Sheldon Glueck since the 1940s, by the early appearance of repeated truancy, fighting in school, and other indicators of social maladjustment.

The character disorders—principally the antisocial personality disorder—are probably exhibited in a majority of the chronic recidivist male prison population in the United States. The psychopath exhibits the typical characteristics of the typical prison inmate: difficulty with impulse control, inability to form lasting relationships, inability to trust others, externalization of difficulties, wish for quick solutions to problems, poor sense of identity, and fear of dependency.

Of the following factors, at least four must be present for a positive diagnosis of antisocial personality disorder: inability to sustain consistent work behavior, inability to function as a responsible parent, failure to accept social norms of behavior, inability to maintain an enduring attachment to a sexual partner, irritability and aggressiveness, failure to honor financial obligations, failure to plan ahead, disregard for the truth, and reckless behavior.

The borderline personality disorder, a relatively newly described entity, is now being identified in some prison systems. Whereas the antisocial personality disorder has a strongly male predominance, the borderline personality has a somewhat female predominance. There is some evidence that the antisocial personality disorder which may have strong hereditary components, appears between the ages of five and fifteen and may even burn out after the age of forty-five.

The condition known as the borderline personality, now an official term in the *DSM*-III, was perhaps first described in 1949 by Hoch and Politin as "pseudo-neurotic schizophrenia." Borderline personality disorder became a recognized disorder in the

1950s and has been well documented (Mack, 1975). A person with a borderline personality has a unique capacity for producing a great deal of anxiety among those taking care of him or her and for getting the various care givers to start fighting among themselves. People with character disorders have difficulty incorporating reality with their affective life. They are people to whom "something is always happening."

Learning disabled persons are usually of at least average intelligence. Nonetheless, for a variety of emotional and, perhaps, genetic and neurologic reasons, some 7 to 15 percent of the general population, and perhaps as many as three-quarters of the male prison population, have serious problems with reading, writing, and learning. The frustration of performing badly in school probably contributes to behavior problems in school, problems that inevitably appear in the records of those people later serving time in prison.

The causes of learning problems are difficult to determine. Some of them may run in families and are more often inherited through the father's side. If this is the case, one would suspect a strong genetic component to learning disabilities. That learning disabilities are four to seven times more common among boys than girls reinforces the notion that genetics must play an important role. Early parental neglect and child abuse, however, are also widely held to be contributing factors and cannot be ignored in discussing the dyslexia and learning disabilities found in prison inmates.

An estimated 75 percent of the long-term inmates show evidence of dyslexia and related deficits of communication. Studies at Patuxent, Maryland, and elsewhere have confirmed this increased incidence, and several programs like the one in Utah to remedy communication deficits have been attempted. To date, there is no evidence that these programs have had an effect or that defects in communication contribute in any way to recidivist criminal behavior.

The most important missing link is our ignorance of any biological relationship between maleness, learning disability, and antisocial personality disorder. It is tempting, but dangerous, to speculate on possible associations. Oversimplification, special pleading, and moral biases have not been helpful in the past and will only continue to obscure the real questions.

Violence

Genes, hormones, learning, and environment all contribute to the tendency of some people to seek violent solutions to a wide range of problems. To this we add the special phenomenon of group violence in which even the most gentle person may become unreasonably savage. The matter of violence is complex and poorly understood. At present there is what might be an artificial distinction between individual violence—which is the domain of psychiatry to treat—and group violence—which has been considered more properly a social phenomenon. Prison riots are the most dramatic (and possibly increasing) manifestations of group violence, and we know little indeed of their dynamics.

Violence is largely a matter of degree. All people apparently have the capacity for violent behavior. In almost everyone there appears to be some sense of delight, almost even ecstasy, in violence. In some contexts—as, for instance, war, sports, verbal encounters, and symbolic representations—violence is acceptable and even praiseworthy. In films, theater, works of art, violence is offered as entertainment. In yet other contexts, however, usually depending on who is acting "violently," those same acts may be punishable by imprisonment or even death.

Violent behavior, with or without assault, is a prime cause for imprisonment and presents both diagnostic and management problems to the prison medical team. Increasing numbers of people in prison are subject to episodes of seemingly uncontrollable violent behavior. Because few mental health facilities in the United States are suitable for the treatment of violent offenders, most hospitals refuse to care for them and they end up in prisons and jails. Most prisons and jails, of course, are poorly equipped and ill-suited to treating violent offenders; isolation and restraint are the best available techniques.

Repetitive violent behavior has been described by Ervin as episodic dyscontrol, with the following features: repeated acts of physical violence, at least three episodes, and actions recognized by peers as inappropriate (Bach-y-Rita et al., 1971).

Objects of the violence can be other persons, self, animals, or physical objects. If the numbers of men in prison exhibiting violent aggressive behavior merely reflect depopulation of the mental hospitals, then it may be that there is a constant amount of this trait, independent of the economy, socialization, or other factors. In support of this, the U.S. Department of Justice reported in 1986 that whereas the rate of convictions for larceny and motor vehicle thefts fell in the period 1973–1984, the incidence of crimes of violence did not change significantly.

To get at the causes of violence, a physician wants to know about the patient's history, neurologic and physiologic status, and living conditions in the prison. The possibility is always present, for instance, that the inmate's violence is a realistic adaptation to the prison situation. Not all people who feel threatened and act out their defensive postures are paranoid; not all paranoids, for that matter, are unthreatened.

In a prison, unlike outside, violence is inevitable and inescapable. When, where, and who are all difficult to predict, but the generally violent atmosphere of prison guarantees that sooner or later someone will erupt. A history of fighting, temper tantrums, school and work truancy, inability to get along with others, as well as a history of self-destructive behaviors can be found in habitually violent inmates. This suggests the likelihood of emotional and perhaps even neurologic bases for the violence.

Social history is also a good index. Violent inmates are likely to have had violent childhoods. In a search for precursors of violent behavior in women in the Framingham (Massachusetts) Prison for Women, investigators found an unusually high incidence of maternal loss before age of ten, a history of excessively severe punishment by parents, and a greater than expected number of blood relatives with organic diseases of the central nervous system. It now appears that excess of male hormones—androgens— may also be a factor.

Abnormalities in the chromosomes of violent offenders may be implicated in violent behavior; but the significance of these chromosomal abnormalities remains to be clarified. A large study still going on in Denmark has found that men with an extra X or Y

chromosome are more likely to be sent to prisons or mental hospitals than men with the normal complement of one X and one Y chromosome; but this finding is not sufficient to determine treatment of those individuals found to have such chromosomal abnormalities. Many people not in prison and not manifesting violent behavior also have X and Y abnormalities.

Other fads and ad hoc theories have suggested quick remedies for criminal violent behavior by medical means. One such fad explanation is the current theory that diet is responsible for deviant behavior. The so-called Twinkie defense in California, in which overconsumption of simple sugars was the explanation of murderous rage, and the anecdotal evidence that reducing simple sugars in the diets of prison inmates reduced aggressive behavior have lent some credibility to the theory. It has not been tested with anything approaching scientific rigor, however.

Treatment

Psychiatric problems are medical problems. The brain is an organ, more complex than most, but perhaps no different in its fundamental biology. The day will probably come, therefore, when the pharmacologic management of psychiatric illness will be as sophisticated and effective as, say, the pharmacologic management of such other chronic illnesses as arthritis or high blood pressure. For now, despite this optimism for the future, resolution of psychiatric problems must depend on behavioral, not pharmacologic, interventions.

The environments of correctional institutions must, above all, be stable. An acutely psychotic inmate creates a crisis. A disruptive inmate therefore presents an intolerable disturbance of the highly prized status quo. Suicide, florid psychosis, and aggressive acting out are therefore likely to be treated as disciplinary problems rather than psychiatric ones. The role of the mental health worker, as a result, often becomes that of disciplinarian, therapist, and health advocate as correctional authorities seek to simplify problems of the inmate's mental and emotional status by labeling him a troublemaker.

The treatment of mental illness within prisons has always been a problem. The institution itself is not conducive to good mental health. Specialized prison mental hospitals do exist but they tend to be used for the criminally insane or for those inmates so violent that they cannot be managed in normal prison settings. In every jurisdiction where they have been investigated, these hospitals for the criminally insane have been criticized severely. The criticism is well founded but unfair. Without adequate funding, staffing, or legal support, workers in such institutions are expected to cope with problems of overwhelming magnitude.

Transferring nonviolent prisoners in whom the risk of escape is low to community mental health facilities has alleviated some of the problems, but results have been inconsistent. Treating mentally disturbed prisoners in community facilities has failed because members of the community in which they are housed fear and distrust the people they see as dangerous criminals. Workers in such institutions do not want to be jailers and resent the constraints imposed on them by the needs for security.

Mental health professionals are usually brought to the prisons to treat emotionally disturbed prisoners. Unlike the clients these mental health workers work with outside, in prisons they must work with groups of hostile, skeptical, and suspicious inmates. Without the therapeutic contract between therapist and client, little can be accomplished. Inmates have little interest in upholding their part of the contract. Consequently, because time, money, and energy are short, rewards are few and hard won, and social and cultural differences between therapists and inmates abound, effective therapeutic communication is all but impossible.

It would appear that in the antitherapeutic environment of the correctional setting, no therapy other than enforced learning of socialization by peer group treatment is effective. Presently accepted methods of psychotherapy seem to be completely ineffective in the treatment of character disorders. According to some experienced correctional authorities and two convicts addressing a 1972 Prison Health Project conference in Boston, the only therapy worth mentioning is group therapy, preferably group therapy led by a peer rather than by an outside authority figure. There is no known pharmacotherapy, and the character disorders do not preclude the coexistence of affective disorders or of schizophrenia. The incidence of alcohol and drug abuse is probably higher in this group than in the general population; although no causal relationship is established or likely.

Finding help for violent offenders is a perpetual problem. A survey of 156 psychiatrists in the Boston area revealed that two-thirds of them would not accept violent patients. The majority of those therapists who did treat violent patients were young, male, and still in their residency training. Even this small group felt that the primary responsibility for preventing violence lay with the patient and the social network rather than with the psychiatrist.

Correctional considerations take legal precedence over medical considerations in the management of violent inmates. In fact, the legal measures may be quite contrary to the therapeutic measures that would otherwise be prescribed. The physician must struggle not to be used by the correctional authorities for their own ends when dealing with a violent inmate. Isolation and seclusion may be therapeutic or punitive; the distinction is sometimes a fine one. Treating the violent offender with such drugs as benzodiazepines and phenothiazines may be indicated by the medical or psychiatric crisis or they may be merely the pharmacologic means of restraining the inmate. Chemical chains are not treatment at all.

These factors are well known and should not be controversial, but violent behavior provokes violent feelings and reason is often overruled by other considerations. As there are many causes of violent behavior, so there are many remedies, reflecting the beliefs of the time. Changes in environment, medication, and psychotherapy can help.

Physicians are accustomed to seeking organic or, at least, psychophysiologic roots to manifest behavioral problems. Temporal lobe epilepsy (now called "complex partial seizures") or other seizure disorders are consequently favorite diagnoses for the underlying cause of repetitive violent behavior. Drugs such as phenytoin (Dilantin) and, as mentioned, psychosurgery are thus perceived as practical and direct solutions to problems of violence. The difficulty is that cases of violent behavior directly attributable to organic brain disease are few, and documented cases of violent behaviors changed for the better by drugs or psychosurgery are even fewer.

MALENESS AND VIOLENT CRIME

A widely publicized book (Wilson and Herrnstein, 1985) marshals evidence that the chronic recidivist or repeating prisoner is a special and distinct type of person from those who commit an isolated crime. Their book raises doubts about the common assumptions that poverty, race, and lack of opportunity are the causes for the criminal behavior of some people. If their thesis is sound, there are biological as well as psychological and sociological roots of criminal behavior. Any such discussion arouses strong feelings, both for and against the prisoner. The number of careful, statistically reliable, objective studies of the biology of the recidivist prisoner is remarkably small.

As we have seen, men outnumber women in the long-term prison population by fifteen or twenty to one— a proportion that is more or less constant throughout the prisons of the United States and Europe. Repetitive violent behavior, the antisocial personality disorder, dyslexia, and crimes of sexual aggression have a heavy male preponderance.

There is a considerable literature on violent behavior. The sources of information vary: courts and correctional organizations, animal biology, endocrinology, neurology, sociology, and, most unfortunately for scientific appraisal, assessments based on ethics and religion. Violence as seen in crimes leading to imprisonment or occurring in prisons themselves is more commonly associated with alcohol than with any other cause. Erving and others have attempted to identify repetitive, relatively unprovoked, aggressive and destructive behavior as episodic dyscontrol syndrome. This condition has been linked with temporal lobe disorders, birth defects, hereditary tendency, and a variety of neurologic disorders under the previously mentioned imprecise but widely used term "chronic brain syndrome." It does appear from the literature, however, that violence that is culturally conditioned, caused by alcohol, PCP, and possibly other substances, and epidemic violence as seen in riots are separate and different from the repeated violence of certain prisoners.

The realization that sexuality, as represented by the male sex hormones, is closely linked to aggressive behavior (in women, perhaps, as well as men), has led to a new approach in the management of violent, aggressive behavior. Behavior modification by desexualizing the violent offender is, today, what tranquilizers and psychotropic drugs were recently, what Freudian insights were supposed to provide not long ago, and what moral compulsion was supposed to accomplish a century ago.

Some twenty-five years ago, it was found that a synthetic hormone, cyproterone acetate (CPA) acted on all of the organs affected by androgens or male sex hormones and suppressed, to a certain extent, pituitary and adrenal gland activity. CPA was first used medically for cancer of the prostate, precocious puberty, hypersexuality, and for some forms of sexual deviance. Twenty years ago, the treatment of hypersexuality commenced in West Germany and then was extensively tried in Israel, then in England, and at present in Canada. When first suggested for criminals, it was thought that to lower the level of sex hormones in men convicted of the paraphilias (abnormal preconditions for full sexual arousal or gratification, as for example, fetishism, transvestitism, zoophilia, pedophilia, exhibitionism, voyeurism, sexual masochism, and sexual sadism) would be helpful. It was believed that the drug would reduce the obsessional thoughts of sexuality, the intensity of the sex drives, and the degree of sexual fantasy. Not long afterward in various centers, interest was aroused in the presence of elevated levels of male sex hormones in those people who had committed acts of aggressive, violent, and assaultive behavior.

As with so many medical treatments, there was first a wave of great enthusiasm and even a few very optimistic reports, including in the United States one from Johns Hopkins Medical School. In the last two or three years, however, several studies have shown that hormone treatment is no panacea and may, in fact, not be helpful. One of the best known and most effective groups studying the effectiveness of hormones in the control of violent and assaultive behavior is the Isaac Gray Center for Psychiatry in the Law at Rush Medical School in Chicago. This is a group of research investigators, clinicians, and psychologists who have done extensive consulting work in jails and prisons. They studied the use of Depo-Provera as a treatment of the paraphilias by giving enough of the drug to reduce the testosterone levels of male volunteers to 25 percent of the pretreatment level. Treated prisoners suffered the side effects of fatigue, weight gain, and flushing. The result, in the treatment of rapists, however, was disappointing. Major studies in Chicago, Baltimore, and Denmark, as well as discussions at the International Conference on Prison Health in Ottawa, 1983, have led to the conclusions that outcomes of hormone treatment are variable and that there is probably a poor correlation of sex drive and androgen levels.

In the past ten years, first in Western Europe, then Great Britain, Canada, and finally the United States, there has been great interest in identifying elevated levels of androgens in males, particularly those convicted of sex crimes and repeated assaultive behavior. A wave of enthusiasm swept westward to be followed by a silence in the literature, confirming the impression that demasculinizing men by means of feminizing hormones has not been helpful in reversing antisocial behavior. We interviewed a number of persons convicted of a variety of serious sexual offenses in the prison in Grendon, Buckinghamshire, England, the prison generally regarded to have the highest staff-to-inmate ratio and the most intensive therapy programs of any prison in the world. Several of the inmates had indeed been subjected to various treatments and echoed the opinion of the medical director of the prison, Dr. Jack Wright, that such programs had no effect on criminal or assaultive behavior, although high-dose estrogen treatment can indeed cut down on the sexual fantasies, frequency of erections and orgasms. One inmate reported to us that after treatment he had indeed lost all sexual desire for women. "But," he continued, "I still hate them and want to kill them."

SUICIDE

Suicide is most common among the newly arrested in lockups and jails—a phenomenon now widely recognized and the subject of much study at all prison health conferences. On the other hand, most reported studies indicate that long-term prisoners commit suicide at a rate lower than that of the general U.S. population of the same age. The remarkable adaptability of human beings to intolerable situations may be the reason, but the answer may equally well be in the personality structure of the recidivist criminal.

Outside prison, guns and pills are the most likely instruments of suicide. In prison, inmates usually hang themselves by a sheet, belt, necktie, or blanket. Violent disturbed inmates may bash their heads or even try to drown themselves in the toilet bowl.

The old notion that successful suicide gives no advance warning is now known to be wrong. One must look closely for suicide attempts in the first three weeks of imprisonment, more among blacks than whites, and especially during the period between 4 P.M. and midnight. Among mentally ill inmates, schizophrenia and alcoholism, as well as depression, increase the likelihood of suicide attempts. Although an occasional review fails to turn up any predictive data, early warning signals are abundantly clear to those who would only look:

• Sudden change from aggressiveness to quiet
• Sudden change from apathy to purposiveness
• Recent loss of a significant person
• Abrupt giving away of treasured possessions
• Change in eating patterns
• History of self-destructive acts
• Recent significant defeat
• Feelings of worthlessness

Given the profound difficulties psychiatrists and inmates already experience in communicating with each other, the psychiatrist is at a great disadvantage in trying to understand and evaluate the emotional distresses of the inmate-patient. In most instances, guards, medics, and nurses are those who identify potential suicides.

In prisons, seclusion is used for a variety of purposes, some punitive and others therapeutic. The distinction is not always clear to the inmate being isolated or to the staff isolating him. The agitated inmate needs isolation in clean, comfortable, quiet quarters, removed as much as possible from the general confusion of prison life. It helps to explain to the inmate and to the guards the realities of the situation. Bland reassurances and denial of the unpleasant realities of prison life only make matters worse.

When seclusion is necessary, it is important to maintain or to increase the inmate's contact with guards, social workers, and medical staff. This is more easily said than done. There is also the ever present risk of encouraging the inmate to be disruptive simply to enjoy the increased attention. An essential standard of prison medicine calls for a member of the medical team to visit each secluded patient daily.

HYPERTENSION

That hypertension is actually less common among prisoners than among the general population has been one of the greatest surprises in studying prison health. The most striking finding in the relatively small number of reliable surveys of prisoner health is that of the infrequency of hypertension among long-term prisoners. This is particularly remarkable when one considers the disproportionate representation of blacks in the prison population.

Studies of the newly imprisoned younger inmates in city and county jails, while still showing a less than expected incidence of hypertension, approximate more closely the average in the outside world. No data are available to compare the blood pressures of habitual criminals before and after incarceration or after release. There is a need to compare their blood pressure with those of siblings and peers not imprisoned. Until such studies are available—and we have been remarkably unsuccessful in persuading anyone to make such a careful study—one can only speculate as to the robustness of the observation and, if the phenomenon is occurring, to the mechanisms. The low incidence of hypertension is not caused by low salt intake or the absence of other factors commonly associated with high blood pressure. Any hypothesis regarding the association of anger and hypertension is disproved by the long-term prison population, a population of men angry by constitution and whose anger is exacerbated by circumstance.

The low incidence of hypertension is much more evident among long-term prisoners than among the newly arrested or those seen in short-term holding jails. The incidence of hypertension was extremely low, for instance, among prisoners in the Deer Island City Prison (Boston) and the long-term maximum-security prison at Norfolk (Massachusetts). The largest and most careful study was reported by Culpepper and Froum (1980). In their survey of 912 inmates in New York State, they found significantly lowered pressures compared to those of the general population. The overall incidence of hypertension among the prison population was 6 percent compared with an estimated 20 percent among the general population. Culpepper and Froum found this low incidence of hypertension to be independent of age, sex, weight, or race.

In another survey of 420 prisoners admitted to New York City correctional facilities in June 1975, Novick and DellaPenna and associates (1975) found the rate of hypertension to be 3.3 percent among men and 10 percent among women. Three groups of inmates were studied in the Tombs Prison in New York City in 1973. There were two groups of 101 and 70 inmates with no hypertension; a third group of 76 inmates had a rate of 9.2 percent. In all groups, the rate of hypertension was far below the national average.

No survey of prison health has noted an unusually high incidence of hypertension. Considering the disproportionately large numbers of blacks in prisons in this country, the low incidence is even more striking. Black people are known to be at high risk for developing hypertension.

A general health survey at the Charles Street Jail (Boston), a holding jail primarily for short-termers, showed a very low incidence of hypertension (Mindlin and Pollack, 1973). As might be expected, inmates with a family history of hypertension were more likely than other prisoners to be hypertensive.

Why is hypertension so uncommon in prison? Possible explanations are the nature of prison life, diet, genetic peculiarities of the prison population, the antisocial personality of most prison inmates, educational level, and length of imprisonment. At this point, no one can explain the unexpected finding (Ostfield, 1987).

Hypertension is almost certainly caused by a combination of

physiological, psychological, genetic, and environmental factors. Learning more about the conditions that determine blood pressure in the prison population may tell us more about the causes of this mysterious disease. At this point there are more questions than answers: What was the blood pressure of these inmates before their imprisonment? What is the family history? What happens to the inmates' blood pressures after they are released from prison? Why do long-term inmates have lower blood pressures than short-term inmates? Does prolonged imprisonment actually lower blood pressure or are long-term inmates so constituted that they simply have lower blood pressures than the general population?

We do not know.

PEPTIC ULCER

Because money, equipment, and staff are insufficient, X-rays (GI series) or gastroscopy are seldom available to prisoners. We have no way of stating categorically the frequency of peptic ulcers and ulcerlike disease. It does appear from a few of the survey reports and from clinical experience that peptic disease is more frequent in prisons than outside.

INFECTIOUS DISEASES WITH ATYPICAL PRESENTATION IN THE PRISON SETTING

Several infectious diseases have atypical presentation in the prison setting. The classical "jailhouse fever" was typhus, which has not been seen in U.S. prisons for many years. Typhoid fever, formerly frequent, now appears infrequently and only then as a homosexually transmitted disease. Malaria, acquired by the use of a shared needle from war veterans who had seen action in Southeast Asia still occurs in prisons, but less frequently than ten years ago. Syphilis does not have an unusually high prevalence, except among some of the newly incarcerated, who occasionally have the highly contagious secondary lesions of skin and mucous membranes. But anal, vaginal, penile, and pharyngeal gonorrhea are frequently seen. Many jail systems now include anal and throat cultures for gonococcus as part of the admissions work-up, and as we have seen, the issue of the right of the prisoners to refuse these tests is unresolved. Riis in Wisconsin and two groups in New York City reported markedly increased prevalence of gonorrhea and trichomonas infections among imprisoned adolescent women.

CONCLUSION

As we have seen, there are remarkably few accurate studies of the presentation of diseases among the inmates of jails and prisons, a substantial group of our population. We have mentioned reasons why these studies have not been conducted. Personality disorders have fallen between enforcement authorities, penologists, and psychiatrists; yet they are responsible for most of the chronic recidivist criminal behavior. The best hope for reducing the increasing numbers of psychopaths in prisons may be in early identification and, if possible, preventive treatment, and yet, we see little progress in this direction. Hypertension, a disease widely studied elsewhere, has a peculiar presentation in the prison population, elucidation of which might make valuable contributions to our knowledge of hypertension inside prisons and out. Here too, progress has been halting and desultory. Control of the AIDS epidemic and of hepatitis B still constitute an unmet public health challenge.

The benefits of such studies are clear. Where common illnesses have a peculiar pressentation among the prison population, study of these unique features may shed light on the basic biologic mechanisms of the disease. Illnesses among prison inmates, whether like or unlike those found outside prisons, still require adequate and careful treatment. Without objective knowledge of what those diseases are, how they present, and how they may best be treated in the prison setting, treatment must suffer. Finally, some diseases (AIDS is a noteworthy example) are much more common within the prison population than in other populations. Studying the disease in this population therefore provides the needed cases and, as important, may eventually offer a means of controlling the disease in one significant segment of the population at risk. After all, inmates are released, in time, back into the general population.

The obstacle to these and other vitally needed medical studies are those placed by prejudice, unwillingness to face unpleasant and low-paid tasks conferring low prestige, and a false sense of economy. At least one study has shown that good prison health care costs less than symptomatic treatment and crisis management. There is need for government at all levels to accept its responsibility for those placed in its custody and for the medical profession to demonstrate its stated desire to render health care to all people. Ignorance of the health status of a million citizens does the profession no credit.

7
Rights and Standards

Health workers in the correctional setting have long been familiar with the profound differences between prison medicine and the practice of medicine elsewhere. Gradually the wider community is recognizing that prison medicine demands rules of procedure and standards unlike those in other medical practices. The environment in which physicians, nurses, and corpsmen must work is wholly unlike most environments in which other health care personnel work. In prison, caring ordinarily takes a distant second place to the perceived and actual demands for physical security. Health care can be given or withheld as reward or punishment. Access to care is always balanced with the threat of breaching security by allowing undue freedom for inmates to come and go.

Moreover, the physical facilities often leave much to be desired. Anywhere else, patients and health care providers would lobby, agitate, and bargain for improvement. In the prison setting, patients have no powerful voice and physicians may be demoralized and politically impotent. The result is often a bad medical situation made all the more serious by a pervasive desire to maintain an uneasy status quo.

Prison health care is made more unlike other health care settings by the thick atmosphere of paranoia. Mutual distrust sours all relationships—those between administrators interested in punishment and health care providers as well as between health care providers and the inmates they care for.

As we have seen, prison medicine differs from most other practice setting in the population it serves. Prison physicians see, for the most part, young, healthy men. A disproportionately high percentage of the men they see are black. The issue of race in criminology remains complex and unresolved. The issue of youth, on the other hand, is clear. Except for the ravages of chronic drug and alcohol abuse, the prison population is generally healthy. In fact, if we consider hypertension (to take a notable example), the prison population is inexplicably *healthier* than the general population and significantly healthier than other young black men.

There has been yet another fundamental difference between how medicine has been practiced in jails and prisons, on the one hand, and how it has been practiced in the rest of society, on the other. Like most other activities behind bars, prison medicine has been practiced behind heavy shrouds of secrecy. Except for occasional exposés and short-lived reform efforts, prison medicine has gone without public scrutiny. It is continued, for the most part, beyond public awareness. Outside of prisons and jails, health care providers and facilities have been inspected, licensed, certified, maintained, and regulated. Within the walls, in sharp contrast, almost anything could go on.

This state of affairs has changed in recent years with the formulation of standards for prison medicine. This has been changed, too, by the enactment of civil rights legislation and regulations to give the professional standards legal standing in court.

Finally, there is the major conflict of *care* and *punishment* that is a fact of life in prison medicine. This central irony colors all health care in jail and prison: the same institution that is responsible for punishing offenders is also responsible for giving them the care they need. At times the dilemma of care and punishment has been resolved in one direction or the other. Recently, with the passage of stronger civil rights legislation in the United States, we have tried to balance the two. In attempting to strike such a balance, however, we have most often merely caught ourselves on the horns of the dilemma.

It is no longer merely a truism of political and social liberals but, in many instances, the law, that prisoners are entitled to the best health care available. The courts have said that this right is guaranteed by the Constitution; it is enforced by several sets of standards written to define the level of health care to which prison inmates are entitled. But, although it is easy to state a right, translating an abstract right into concrete action has proved difficult indeed.

Inmates have violated the acceptable rules of behavior. They are placed in institutions as punishment. The courts have decreed that there be no cruel and unusual punishment and that denial of access to adequate medical care is, in fact, cruel and unusual punishment. Nowhere have court decisions or class action suits guaranteed improvement, correction, or reform of the individual. The term "care" is used loosely. To the law, this is essentially a parental or custodial function. To the patient, care means warmth, sympathy, and compassion. Standards can insure everything but these intangible, yet necessary, aspects of adequate medical care. Society has not been able to legislate warmth and compassion and probably most citizens feel no necessity to supply these to prison inmates. Yet there is almost inevitable in Western society a feeling of discomfort about their absence from the prison medical scene. The right to medical care, both in and out of prison, can only mean access to an acceptable level of care. Critics of prison health care say that the inmates are asking for bread and have been given only a stone. Establishing and implementing standards has sharpened the issue of care versus punishment.

Translating abstract right to action has been made even more difficult by the common understanding that prison inmates are entitled to something better than adequate care. Some advocates maintain that prison and jail inmates are entitled to the *best* medical care available. The justification for this entitlement is that by virtue of severely limiting an inmate's personal freedom, the federal, state, or local government assumes the *obligation* to provide the best services it can find. More moderate observers of prison health care hold that inmates are entitled to the level of medical care practiced in the community outside.

The concept of a right to the best medical care available is difficult for several reasons. First, the concept of "best care" is itself unclear and this obscurity is deepened by our confusion about "right." Ever since rights became divorced from divinity, the line between right and political expediency has become blurred by realities of the real world. Arguments of a right to health care either founder in metaphysics or get lost in politics. Second, interpretations of the constitutional right to adequate and more-than-adequate health care change with the times. Finally, it is almost impossible to define what might be "the best health care" for prison and jail inmates or for anyone else, for that matter, because people's perceptions of health and expectations of care differ so sharply. Assigning relative values to personal caring, professional competence, and accessibility of inmates to care is difficult at best and may well be impossible.

The Englishman John Howard (1726–1790) and the Italian Cesare Bonesana Beccaria (1738–1794) began the "reform" process that continues to this day of codifying the obligations of prison authorities and the rights of prison inmates, especially rights to health and safety. Beccaria's treatise, *Dei delitti e delle pene* was written in 1764. In eighteen months the book went through six editions; it was eventually translated into twenty-two European languages. John Howard's early statement of the rights of prisoners, *The State of Prisons*, likewise was influential from the time of its publication in 1777.

Howard's proposed standards, which were incorporated in the model regulations for health care at Shrewsbury in 1794, have a surprisingly modern ring. He called for a daily visit to the prison by a physician, a complete physical examination of each prisoner on admission, and the requirement that the prison physician see each inmate at least once a week. Furthermore, Howard required justices of the peace to inspect jails to see that the walls and ceilings were scraped and whitewashed annually, that the rooms were cleaned and ventilated, that infirmaries were established to care for the sick and inform inmates, that adequate clothing was distributed to the inmates, and that the dungeon was used as infrequently as possible.

More than two hundred years later, the recommendations by Beccaria and Howard for the humane governance of jails and prisons are still regarded by some as unenforceable in statute and idealistic almost to the point of fantasies. One clear problem is that it has proved difficult indeed to establish standards of cleanliness, personal and public hygiene, and medical attention.

At one end of the scale, there are occasional spasms of public outrage at the mistreatment of inmates in jails and prisons. At the other end of the scale, there is public outcry about so-called Cadillac medicine being inappropriate within the walls of correctional institutions.

Dr. Kerr White, dean of the Johns Hopkins School of Public Health, described in 1967 the five Ds representing those things that a proper health care system is supposed to prevent—death, disease, disability, discomfort, and dissatisfaction. No one can argue about the first three and, to a certain extent, these are matters of technology, knowledge, and facilities. Discomfort and dissatisfaction, on the other hand, are the most important for the patient, the least involved in technology, and require the most subjective judgment. Even the best physicians under the best circumstances cannot prevent discomfort wholly, although they can sometimes relieve acute pain to some degree. As for dissatisfaction, this is largely a function of the outcome of the illness, over which the physician has less control than most people would like to believe.

In the best-run prison health facilities, the five Ds can be managed almost as well as in the civilian world. In some respects, as we have seen in the chapter on the management of illness in prisons, better; for the jail setting gives a measure of control over patient's lives that some physicians who treat people in the outside world would envy.

The question of standards is of historical and practical importance. Historically, the development of standards represents the growing attitude on the part of correctional authorities, medical staff, and the courts that health care in the prison setting must be made more rational. In the absence of written standards, for instance, the system is always vulnerable to special pleading by the inmates. As we have seen, complaints about inadequate health care and then demands for changes are a regular feature of prison unrest. The practical benefit of having written standards is that law, medicine, corrections, press, public observers, and inmates all have joined, more or less, in consensus of what the minimum medical services should be.

In setting standards, the problem remains of whether the standards should establish a floor or a ceiling. Standards could spell out in detail an operational definition of "the best" medical care or they could establish a tolerable minimum. Until recently, the standards were written more in the spirit of the former. They set forth clearly what services were the legitimate expectations of patients and providers. More recently, in line with changes throughout medicine, the notion of prison medicine has shifted toward that of effective minimum (although it is never called that) in the interests of cost containment and appropriate allocation of finite medical resources. As health maintenance organizations have burgeoned in the society outside jails, so efforts to contain costs within jails have also been redoubled.

The development of standards put prison health on the road toward a more businesslike system. Once this reform was accomplished, the next logical step, of which we are beginning to see signs, is the provision of health care services strictly as a business (see chapter 4). A result is that planning health care in or out of prisons must resolve three powerful forces—right to care, acceptable standards of care, and cost.

HOW RIGHTS BECAME STANDARDS

One of the dilemmas of life is how to square reality with ideals, and how to make what *is* in life approach what we believe *ought to be*. This dilemma is even more painful when dealing with prisons and prisoners because there is no agreement as to the goals or ideals. Those who think they know the realities and the realistic possibilities evidently march to a drummer different from the one the theorists and moralists hear. For many years, in Massachusetts for at least eighty years, regulations and standards have been established by legislation or by executive order specifying minimum requirements for the Department of Correction in regard to sanitation, food, exercise, and access to medical care. These standards are generally attainable, although for a variety of reasons they are difficult to meet. The jails or prisons not meeting them might reasonably expect enforced remedial or even punitive action. Such actions were rarely, if ever, taken before the 1970s when the political and social climate urged profound changes in many social institutions. Prior to that time, there was no political or popular base for prison systems to try to make their facilities conform with the existing standards.

In 1970, the American Nursing Association recognized prison health care as a special field of interest and drew up a pioneering statement of standards to be maintained. In 1973, the American Medical Association and the American Bar Association jointly published a compilation of standards, including those from the United Nations, the American Correctional Association, the National Sheriffs Association, the Federal Bureau of Prisons, and those of many states. The outlines of these standards are generally similar. Throughout the 1970s, these standards were extended to represent hopes or theories rather than minimum levels strictly related to physical health. Standards were augmented, for instance, to require at least one full-time psychiatrist for each prison, in the expressed hope that prison psychotherapy would cure deviant behavior. Other sets of standards and recommendations made the uncontradicted statement that good health practices would prevent recidivism. These untested assumptions remind us of the eighteenth- and nineteenth-century hopes for the rehabilitative effects of religious and moral treatment of prisoners. That groundless optimism was transformed to twentieth-century hopes for the remedial effects of prison health care.

RIGHTS, CONSENSUS, STANDARDS, CONTRACTS

Before we go any further, we must pause for definitions of some key terms. Right, consensus, standards, and contracts are large legal abstractions on which the practical details of daily life are based. Ordinarily, they go unquestioned. In the matter of prison medicine, however, they are almost constantly questioned and require redefinition and reaffirmation as social and political attitudes shift.

The word *right* has two somewhat different senses. In the abstract, it means the moral principles that form the basis of justice and guarantee the ethical content of laws. As a definition, this may not help much, however, for it replaces the one abstraction *right* with two others, *justice* and *ethics*, which are no easier to define. In its concrete sense, the word *right* connotes the powers, privileges, and demands one person can make upon another person. In a strictly legal sense, right is defined as "a capacity residing in one man of controlling, with the assent and assistance of the state, the actions of others." Right is what one person can expect to receive of another, simply by virtue of being a human being. These are so-called natural rights. Civil rights belong to every member of a community by virtue of being a member of that community.

This, however, is where the trouble lies. The line between natural right and civil right is not clear, and the moral and ethical basis of civil right is ultimately natural right. Consequently, the operational basis of decision on the adequacy of health care in prisons has been *consensus*. A consensual contract has been made in the past, based on civil law, in which obligations to provide adequate medical services have been established without any external formalities or other symbolic act to bind the contract.

The *standard* by which adequacy has been judged, has been essentially the standard of what "a reasonable man under like circumstances" would do. Legal definitions of standards are based on the general recognition of and conformity to established practice.

When standards are negotiated and written down as concrete guidelines for action, they become the basis of a contract. A *contract* is a promissory agreement between persons that creates a legal relation; the terms and conditions are clear and the penalties for failing to honor those terms and conditions are likewise clear. The better the contract, the stronger the relationship.

Standards represent objective measures which have had notable success in improving medical care, both inside the prisons and out. In the outside world, competition, monetary rewards, and penalties have led to minimum levels of conformity. In prisons and jails, standards have led to litigation. Those in charge of health care can both thank and blame the lawyers.

The greatest change originated within the health profession itself. A group of nurses led by Rena Murtha, then of the New York City prison health system, persuaded the American Nursing Association at its 1973 annual meeting to declare as a policy that adequate health care of prisoners was a right. Within the American Public Health Association a year or so later, physicians from the New York City system and San Francisco formed a group which met regularly, wrote standards for health care, and proposed implementing these standards by means of a process of inspection and accreditation.

Accreditation became a fact in 1975 when the American Medical Association, with the help of support and money from the federal Law Enforcement Assistance Administration (LEAA), started inspecting jails and established comprehensive standards with procedures for evaluation and certification for those jails that were successful. As of January 1988, 282 jails, prisons, and juvenile facilities have been accredited. To date, however, fewer major state and federal prisons and no correctional mental health facilities have been subjected to this procedure, although standards are in place. The fear of failure to meet these standards clearly deters institutions from participating in accreditation programs.

These standards evidently protect the jail system. A startling proof of this is the fact that no jail that has been accredited is at present under law suit. In 1984, however, approximately 20 percent of all other jails and prisons in the United States were under court order or suit. This does not necessarily prove that the standards are correct, but it shows that they fit in with the majority legal and social opinions of this time.

When we start to examine more closely the reasons for these standards, we increasingly run into the assumption that adequate health care is a right. Rights are declared by human beings, not handed down from above. Nor are they encoded in our genes. Life, liberty, and the pursuit of happiness seem to be accepted as rights in the Western world. Rights and the standards that derive from them actually represent a consensus of the social attitudes of law, medicine, the press, legislature, and the clergy. The advantage of consensus is that it protects against special pleading and unlimited demands. Some rights have been stated but no effort made to implement them because it probably would be impossible to guarantee them. Everyone, for example, would probably agree that we share a right to breathe unpolluted air, to eat uncontaminated food, to have sufficient food, and to enjoy the comforts and security of an adequate shelter and clothing. It would be most unfashionable to deny that these are rights. It is curious that in the United States these rights are only in part translated into systematic and well-financed actions. The right to medical care, on the other hand, has been translated into action in almost every country of the world.

In summary, rights represent a consensus view. Standards are established to put flesh on the abstract bones of rights. The law acts to enforce standards. When these standards are strictly defined and capable of solution, the system seems to work. When attempts are made to impose views outside of the consensus, trouble begins. For example, some have tried to make a low-carbohydrate diet as standard in prisons on the theory that nutritional changes can modify violent behavior. Others wish to compel endocrine evaluation and compulsory treatment for those convicted of sex crimes and other assaultive behavior. Still others would mandate sex education, health counseling, dental hygiene, and a host of other special programs to which, in their words, prison inmates are "entitled."

EXPRESSED GOALS AND PRACTICAL STANDARDS

The Criminal Appeals Bureau of the Legal Aid Society of the City of New York published a report of its Prisoners' Rights Project in 1983, including an index of cases and legal memos concerning prisoner medical care (1977–1983). The document is extremely useful and has served as the basis of much that follows in this chapter. Although we will not follow its subject classification, the report is a convenient introduction to the breadth of subjects covered by legal cases and by standards of prison health care (almost all of these have been seen before in various commission reports and in the AMA standards):

- Coverage by physicians and nurses
- Communication of medical needs, including sick call
- Access to outside services, including emergency care, follow-up on appointments, access to specialized care, and so forth

- Access to an inmate's own physician
- Examinations
- Medication
- Qualifications of medical personnel
- Dental care
- Eye care
- Special diets
- Suicide prevention
- Psychiatric services and the rights of the mentally ill
- Drug dependency treatment
- Physical facilities
- Quarantine
- Standards of liability
- Medical records

A brief survey of some cases covered in this list will give a good idea of the complexity of medical-legal problems in the jails and prisons. One of the most notable qualities of these cases is their peculiar admixture of pathetic, tragic, and trivial concerns. In many cases, the ultimate disposition of the court is less interesting than the fact that the case was submitted to court in the first place.

For example, *Porter* v. *Windham* (Oklahoma, 1981) found that the failure of the jail to provide safety shoes and prevent recurrence of foot fungus did not constitute a legitimate claim. *Grubb* v. *Bradley* (Tennessee, 1982) likewise found that lack of centralized authority in the medical care system, absence of system-wide health care policies and protocols, lack of continuity of care, failure to provide prescribed medications, failure to provide adequate protection against the outbreak of communicable diseases, poorly organized pharmacy services, housing of healthy inmates in hospital beds, improper storage of medication, and delays in sick call did not violate constitutional provisions. *Venus* v. *Goodman* (Wisconsin, 1983) is based on a claim for deprivation of medical care and a malpractice suit, claiming "deliberate indifference" to the inmate's medical condition in refusing to give him less demanding work assignments and in delaying referral to a specialist. *Wellons* v. *Townley* (Virginia, 1981) found that a dentist's refusal to prescribe addtional medication for pain did not violate constitutional guarantees; but *Daniels* v. *Murphy* (Oklahoma, 1978) did find a violation of the Constitution when officials lost an inmate's Sinequan pills and refused to get a prescription refilled.

Many of the cases are matters of judgment. In *Sturts* v. *City of Philadelphia* (Pennsylvania, 1982), the plaintiff claimed that the failure to remove stitches promptly, resulting in scarring, was "so woefully inadequate as to amount to no treatment at all."

According to a 1983 Boston presentation by Lynn J. Lund, then inspector general of the Utah State Department of Corrections, there are five key concepts in prison rights:

1. There is a single standard of liability under the federal Civil Rights Act. Consequently, regardless of the size of the correctional facility, there is a legal imperative to meet the standards. The state of Texas has fought the standards; but a $1.6 million ruling by the Fifth Circuit Court of Appeal went against Texas.

2. Budgetary defense is invalid according to the federal court. In several cases, departments of correction have been told that if they cannot provide adequate health care and health facilities, they should not incarcerate people. In Florida, for example, this principle has prompted law enforcement officials not to imprison convicted felons.

3. Documentation is the sine qua non of any case. According to the Supreme Court, if the department of correction cannot provide convincing records that actions were taken, in the eyes of the court, they were not taken.

4. Individuals and departments can be held liable. Liability can be *official*, in which case the employer pays, or it can be *personal*, in which case the individual health care provider pays punitive damages.

5. The principal test, under law, is "deliberate indifference to serious medical needs" (established in *Estelle* v. *Gamble*). "Deliberate indifference" means, in this context, failure to allow the inmate access to diagnostic or therapeutic attention, either because the inmate has been prevented from making his medical condition known or because the corrections authorities have prevented the inmate from getting the attention he needs. "Serious medical needs" have been defined in

the courts as medical conditions that have been diagnosed by a physician or "so obvious that even a lay person would easily recognize the necessity for a doctor's attention." Among serious medical needs are emotional as well as physical needs.

It is not necessary to demonstrate malicious intent to win a judgment. In the case *Smith* v. *Wade* (103 S. Ct. 1625, 1983), an inmate at the Algoa Youthful First Offenders Camp in Missouri was harrassed and sexually assaulted by his two cellmates. Wade won his suit against Smith (compensatory damages $25,000 and punitive damages $5,000) on the argument that even though Smith was not malicious, he should have known what was occurring in Wade's cell and should have moved him to another cell. In other words, it was Smith's "affirmative duty" to guarantee Wade's constitutional rights to health and safety.

The problem, of course, is that "deliberate indifference" and "callous indifference" to the condition of the inmate are complex notions, and to some extent, they depend on what we might call the conscience of society at the time. To establish in court deliberate indifference, it is necessary to show (1) that the defendant knew or should have known what was occurring; (2) a pattern of gross abuse; (3) that nothing was done to remedy a pattern of gross abuse; (4) that preparation for the possibility of such abuse was inadequate (as in the case of a single brutal incident coming as the result of inadequate training).

STANDARDS

While the line separating correctional, security, and health care considerations is difficult to draw in relation to standards, the distinction must be made if we are finally to divorce the health care of inmates from matters of moralizing or philosophizing. As we have seen, these moral and philosophic concerns vary from time to time and from place to place. The American Correctional Association has had for years a very good jail and prison accreditation program (part of which involves jail and prison health). Health concerns are included with disciplinary and administrative considerations.

Standards developed by the American Medical Association, and now being carried on by the National Commission on Correctional Health Care (NCCHC), are confined to matters of reasonable and generally acceptable standards of health care. Since their first publication in 1979, they have not been seriously challenged and are likely to be the criteria for many years to come.

Three sets of standards have been published by the commission: (1) First are standards for jails, most recently revised in 1987. On the basis of these standards, some 800 jails have been inspected, accredited, and reviewed. (2) The standards for prisons in July 1979 (revised 1987), have been implemented more slowly for the acknowledged reason that few large prison systems could be expected to pass without drastic increase in procedure and expenditure. (3) The standards for juvenile facilities, first published in August 1979, were revised in August 1984. They have been checked, audited, and discussed many times and not seriously challenged, although they have not yet been widely implemented.

The NCCHC has not issued standards for correctional mental health facilities. The American Psychiatric Association has been grappling with this problem for some time but has not been able to agree on generally acceptable standards to be published with APA approval.

An illustration of the difficulty of keeping philosophy and moralizing out of strictly health standards is seen if one looks at them closely. There are sixty-nine standards for prisons, fifty-six for jails, and sixty for juvenile facilities. These numbers have stayed fairly constant through the processes of review and revision. Roughly one-third of these standards are considered essential; failure to comply with them results, without question, in the failure to be accredited. The rest are considered important and something approaching 70 percent of these criteria must be met for an institution to be accredited. As a result, there is a certain amount of flexibility and bargaining in the accrediting process.

Looking at the issue of caring, that is, going beyond the mechanical provision of facilities and services, we see reference to "the treatment philosophy." The 1987 NCCHC document says, "Written policy [states] that health care is rendered with consideration of the patient's dignity and feelings." This philosophy asserts the need for privacy during the physical examination of patient inmates and that "verbal permission" from both adult and juvenile inmate patients must be sought before any rectal or vaginal examination is performed. The violent assaultive nature of many inmates and the overriding considerations for security make it virtually impossible, in most institutions, for there to be complete privacy during the examination. For the protection of the health workers, this is perhaps a practical impossibility. The ambiguity here may be sidestepped by the phrase "rendered with consideration" of the patient's dignity and feelings. Perhaps that is as close as one can come.

More telling, in examining the conflict of practical realities and idealized possibilities in the standards and regulations concerning health care in prisons, we often come upon rhetoric, as here, supporting the "dignity and feelings" of the prison inmate-patient. The phrase itself betrays a kind of confusion in the minds of the framers of the standards; for, despite the degree of caring reflected in the phrase, the practical realities of prison medicine make it more than likely that dignity and feelings are among the first considerations to be abandoned as security, sheer expediency, and other concerns gain in importance. Dignity and feelings of inmates were not highly regarded by the society that sought their incarceration.

Again, when the standards described the basic requirements for exercise, they stipulated that a good exercise facility be available for one hour a day, every day (modified in 1987 to three days a week). Nowhere is it stated, however, that the inmate should be compelled to have this exercise, which clearly was not the daily habit of most of the inmates before incarceration. Is there a remnant here of the "muscular Christianity" of the last century, where daily exercise was thought to encourage self-discipline and pure thoughts?

The standards note that bathing and shaving facilities must be provided. Again, the issue of whether inmates can be forced to use them, however, remains open in the standards.

Correctional authorities and visitors to prisons and jails seem always to be impressed by and comforted by cleanliness and neatness. One might ask whether the bathing and exercising are really instituted for the purpose of making the visitors feel better or the prisoners.

In one respect, things have not changed very much in two hundred years. John Howard's recommendations and the standards of 1979 are remarkably similar. In fact, depending on the size of the institution covered by the present standards, physicians may actually be required to make fewer calls than required by Howard's recommendations, put into effect in 1794.

SITE VISIT

The essential feature of the entire process of accreditation and the application of jail standards is, of course, the site visit to the institution. One thing, clear to the National Commission and the correctional authorities, is not very clear to the casual visitor and certainly not to the lay public: rehabilitation of prisoners, desirable as that might be or even remedies for shortcomings of the criminal justice system are not the goal of the NCCHC site visit. The goal of the visit is to insure that a decent, civilized system of medical care conforms to the law.

It is worth looking at what happens on a site visit, for when we send an inspecting team to visit a jail, we are in actuality holding a mirror up to ourselves. We are examining the jail but the blinders and magnifying lenses (as well as the particular distorting lenses) are upon our own eyes.

A jail applies for accreditation to the National Commission on Correctional Health Care, usually after pressure from a court or the local medical society. Various forms are exchanged. A preliminary questionnaire is filled out. The visitors to the jail already have some background information as well as, possibly, some preconceptions. For those who have never been on a visit or have never even been inside a correctional institution, there is a mixture of fear, excitement, and anticipation. The first impression is almost invariably one of the grim, sterile, but neat and clean institution, quiet, and showing all the features we have described in the chapter on the environment.

Not all jails are alike, however, and they can give somewhat different impressions. For example, in the Essex County Jail (Salem, Massachusetts), the cornerstone is marked 1813. The building was erected by captured British sailors. Moves have been made to replace this jail for 150 years, but no other community in the county will hear of relocating the jail near them. As a result, the present Essex County Jail is old and battered, with inadequate plumbing and substandard electrical wiring. In fact, at the time one of us visited it, the women's section of the jail had so little electricity available that only a single 25-watt bulb could be allowed in each cell without blowing the fuses. The women, at the time of one of our visits, had no running water, but used a slop bucket at night exactly as inhabitants of that building had done in 1813.

To give a sense of the complexity of the accrediting process and its goals, however, we must take note of the interesting fact that when the women housed in this Essex County Jail were given the opportunity to relocate to the relatively new, much more spacious, lower security women's prison forty miles away, they all refused. They liked the homey atmosphere of their present house of detention, the intimacy of the guards, access to their families, and perhaps other factors that were not immediately apparent.

The jail at Edgartown, Massachusetts, to give the other extreme, appears from the front of the building to be a typical sea captain's white-painted house. Only when entering the building from the rear is one aware that this is, indeed, a correctional institution. There are only a few prisoners in the jail at any time, all of whom are extremely well cared for and well known to the jailer and the jailer's family. The feeling of family is heightened by the fact that the jailer's wife, who is an excellent cook, merely unlocks the back door of her kitchen at mealtime and brings to the prisoners the same meal that she is preparing for her own family, eating in the front portion of the building.

These two examples will give a clear sense of how difficult it might be to devise uniform standards by which to judge human issues—including those of health—in jails and prisons.

When considering the delivery of good quality medical care in the Charles Street Suffolk County Jail (Boston, Massachusetts), an ancient but handsome and imposing granite structure, one need only look over the wall, across a very narrow street, to the Massachusetts General Hospital, one of the nation's most prestigious medical centers. The 400 inmates at the Charles Street Jail, however, get their medical care from their own physician and nurses. If they require outside consultation for difficult cases, inmates must be transported through dense city traffic from the jail to Boston City Hospital, which is about two miles away.

Some jail staffs receive an inspecting team warmly; others with open suspicion and hostility. Reasons for welcoming the inspection are easy to discern. Accreditation can help a jail negotiate its future budgets, either as a reward for a job well done or, more often, in recognition of outside disapprobation of how things are being done at the jail. Stated somewhat differently, having an accreditation seems to protect jails from legal action if inmates or their representatives seek to bring an action against them.

In other institutions, it is clear that the person who is ostensibly in charge of the medical care is, in fact, a figurehead and the real heart of the operation is a nurse or physician's assistant of great talent. The physician may see a reported forty men a day, but the ongoing medical presence at the jail is the head nurse. She (usually but not always a woman) is the chief administrator and health care provider at the infirmary.

Despite the outward similarities in all jails and prisons, the atmosphere is sometimes strikingly different from one institution to another. One inmate, a federal prisoner who had been involved in the "French connection," was being held in one of the Massachusetts prisons for his own protection. He reported, firsthand, on the remarkably different atmospheres jails can have. He thought he detected national differences. In Spain, he said, the jail was a small institution where conjugal visits were easy to arrange and the cooking was done by the warden's wife. He thought the jail was not very clean, perhaps, but was a "highly civilized place to live." When he was transferred to Switzerland, he found the jail extremely clean and well maintained. All meals, exercise, and other activities were ordered punctually and the behavior of the guards to the inmates was always correct. The Swiss jails, he said, were "almost unbearable." The Massachusetts prison he was in at that time, he felt, was a compromise between the two.

Taking the differences into consideration, it is not surprising that the inspection reports are not always consistent with each other or with other people's impressions of the institutions. The inspecting team has a varied agenda. The first task is probably to decide who is being served. Is the inspection a favor to the National Commission on Correctional Health Care? Is the team to serve as a citizen review committee to see that those who are incarcerated receive fair treatment? Is the team to check on the operations of the Department of Correction? Or is the report in fact, to help secure outside support and backing for the Department of Correction? Is the team to support the jail staff or to be critical of their activities? Is the inspection for the benefit of the inmates, in which the site visit team serves as ombudsmen or advocates for the inmates, or is it as representatives of society to carry out parental responsibilities over those who have lost their civil rights?

The physicians, nurses, and laypeople who serve on the site visit committee interview a number of people in the institution and undertake a rather detailed examination of certain features described in the extensive statement of standards.

Standards for jail health care read very well. They have been thought out carefully and they have been tested. Hearing the statistics on the good results in jails which have been accredited and attending national conferences on correctional health give, perhaps, a false idea of the conflicting emotions, struggles of personalities, and ambiguous findings that are part of any site visit. Standards are distinct and specific, but the people who deliver the health care and their evaluators are human beings with strong feelings and differing emotional agenda. If we work through an accreditation visit to a jail, looking at the various steps and events, the picture may become more vivid, if not more clear-cut.

Prior to the site visit, a lengthy questionnaire prepared by the NCCHC is sent to the institution, to be filled out severally by the physicians, nurses, medical librarian, and other appropriate personnel. NCCHC personnel in Chicago receive and review the material and forward it to the inspecting team selected by the local medical society.

The inspection team almost always includes one or two physicians and nurses, as well as other medical and health care professionals, and sometimes a clerical representative of the medical society who has had experience with this process. The team generally has a balance of experienced observers and new ones who are making their first visit to a jail. These newcomers almost invariably find the inspection tour a profoundly moving—and often disturbing—experience. We remind each observer that he or she is to confine observations, questions, and remarks strictly to the business of the visit, but, being human, the observers often stray from the prescribed questions.

Usually the staff of the jail anticipate the visit with a mixture of pleasant expectation and dread. The themes we have so often mentioned of being misunderstood by the outside world, of being criticized unfairly, and of feeling generally defensive all come to the fore at the time of site visit. It is not surprising, therefore, that sometimes the observer, trying to ask the question listed on the survey form in a neutral manner, is answered with unexpected anger at being interrogated, defensiveness in explaining why some things are just impossible, and a clear unwillingness to participate in the information-gathering process.

The observer talking with an inmate, on the other hand, often finds an unexpectedly willing participant who, for his or her own reasons, may either be full of extreme praise for the health care establishment or extreme condemnation. The observer who does not know the person has no way of checking the validity of the report. Other inmates have refused to be selected or, wishing to be selected, have failed to be admitted to the process. One wonders whether an altogether different set of comments and observations would be the result if the selection of inmates were random.

In any event, the visit goes on usually for the better part of a day, sometimes continuing into a second day. The person in charge of the paper work for the medical society then collects the answers and makes a summary statement that is sent off to Chicago, to the offices of the NCCHC for appraisal. Generally there is correspondence back and forth about the inevitable deficiencies in the reporting process.

The final report frequently seems to be bent slightly in favor of the jail; one cannot help being sympathetic with the efforts of these people to provide care and custody. Criticism, however, sometimes provokes extremely heated responses. At this point, the NCCHC seems almost always to share a bias in favor of accreditation. When some of the essential standards have not been met, members of the NCCHC often suggest ways for the local medical society to exhort, encourage, and, failing that route, compromise.

Whatever the potential shortcomings of this method, it is far superior to any that have previously been in existence. The results, at present, seem to satisfy everyone. The only possible exceptions to this statement are those who earnestly feel that any form of imprisonment is an outrage, and that any reform that tries to ameliorate prison life is a moral evasion.

Accreditation is awarded for one or two years, depending on the circumstances. The certificate itself is generally awarded by an official of the medical society. At the award ceremony, are the sheriff, the jail physician, and an official of the medical society, and perhaps others of the jail health care team, dressed up and smiling as the certificate is handed over. The certification represents a nonjudgmental fulfillment of the standards of decency and the law. Whether or not this has anything to do with rehabilitation or prison reform is entirely beside the point.

Those whose jail could not pass the accreditation or who did not ask for inspection for fear of failure can be heard at district medical society meetings or in the back rows of the section meetings of the annual conferences on jail and prison health. They feel that their earnest efforts have not been rewarded and that they have been criticized for being unable to meet standards which, under their particular circumstances, they felt were impossible.

Some members of the medical society committee, including us, have from time to time felt the discomfort of being caught in the middle of this sometimes seemingly insoluble dilemma. Not only are we involved in care versus punishment of the inmate, but in the process of carrying out a site visit, we have been involved in the issue of support versus punishment of the jail health physician.

SIC TRANSIT REFORM

Reform has given way to the more orderly processes of devising standards of adequate professional behavior in correctional institutions, professional inspection to ascertain that those standards are being met, and litigation in the judicial system when those standards are not met. The impulses behind the reform movements of the early 1970s, of which the Prison Health Project in Massachusetts may well be a prime example, were probably more heartfelt than the impulses motivating reforms of the 1980s. As so often proves to be the case, however, good intentions are not sufficient to win the day.

We are a government of laws not men precisely because of the frailty, confusion, and imperfectability—if we can use such a word—of human beings. Reform, no less than other institutional solutions to human problems, relies on the common human talents and desires, but it is also usually undone by them as well. The goal, therefore, is to construct a system that is workable, that meets the minimum standards arrived at by consensus, and that will work and survive without regard to the selection of superior men and women.

We cannot reasonably expect to have a heroic and superior person in every prison health system. A professor of criminology at the University of Oslo has written that the only solution is to construct systems that can be operated by mediocre people: "Most people are mediocre, and they don't know this." He goes on to say, "Extremely good psychiatrists are often particularly dangerous because we trust them when they say something can be done. We forget that behind them are 35 others who are not so good" (Christie, 1972, p. 161).

Now that the courts have the means of passing judgment on the jails and prisons within their jurisdiction, there is evidence that they are becoming impatient with the slow progress toward reform. Moreover, with half a million people in prison and with professional health care workers taking less than an active interest in prison medicine, the federal courts are seeing themselves increasingly as the only active advocate for prison health care. As a result, federal courts have forced governments to provide resources, staff, programs of health care, and other improvements to bring the correctional institution into conformity with standards already promulgated.

Afterword

Much as we would like to call this closing section of *Care and Punishment* a conclusion, we cannot. If we will learn anything at all from the history of prison health care, it is that there are no ultimate solutions to the problems, only provisional next steps. The political, moral, and scientific certainties of one generation inevitably are rejected by the next. Unfortunately, because the institutions themselves have such short memories, past successes as well as failures seem to have little effect on present decisions. Each generation invents its own more or less effective programs for dealing with crime and for coping with the day-to-day management of prisons that house the men and women criminals.

We would consider this book to have been successful if we conveyed no other information than the need to strengthen the institutional memory. Reasons for institutional amnesia are easy to discern: first and foremost, the topics are painful and unpleasant to consider; the burnout rate is high; and the general oversight is sporadic and often superficial. Moreover, the major interested parties on either side of the wall are often locked into what they see as adversarial relations, a situation that can only feed the paranoia of the correctional side and the self-righteous (often self-serving) outrage of the occasional public servants, journalists, and would-be reformers on the other side.

Our society would be fortunate, indeed, if we enjoyed a moral and ethical consensus on right and wrong. It is always reassuring to appeal to absolutes when confronted by complex, ambiguous, and unresolvable problems. But no such philosophic consensus is available to us. Whether absolute moral truths can be determined at all, by whatever means, we leave to the clergy and professors of ethics. We note only that, to date, no society seems to have been able to dissociate its values from the social and political contexts in which they are applied; and situations are shifty ground on which to base absolute judgments. In short, we are left with great timeless problems but only limited and temporal solutions. We do the best we can.

The ethical issues are not merely academic, however. Crime is a national problem of growing dimensions. The population of prison inmates in the United States is now greater than the population of Denver, Seattle, or St. Louis. The prison population is now about 500,000 and is growing by at least 26,000 annually. More than one million people are sent to jails and prisons each year.

Many people have concluded that, aside from the initial cost to society of the crime itself, punishment of criminals is itself a large and ongoing social cost. To house a person in jail for one year cost an average of $16,000 in 1987. In some states, it costs much more. The total cost to the nation is about $8 billion annually. New prison construction in the United States costs about $50,000 per bed. Just to pay for new construction to house the 26,000 growth in the prison population will cost at least $1.3 billion, and then caring for and feeding this increase will cost another $420 million each year.

"Lock the criminals up" is the recommendation from the highest law enforcement officers in the United States as well as from the man and woman in the street. Like most popular solutions, however, the chief appeal of "Lock them up" is its simplicity. Like most simple solutions to complex problems, it is limited at best and wrongheaded at worst. It is clear, on reflection, that incarcerating this huge population of prison inmates does not deter crime and, moreover, creates its own problems of managing the institutions in which convicts are housed. We can leave aside for the moment questions of what might be the real function of a prison. At this point, we are concerned only with the question of how to provide the services required by such a major city behind bars in our nation. "Crime on the streets" has now been replaced, in the national press, by "overcrowding in prisons" as the main focus of attention.

WHAT HAVE WE LEARNED ABOUT PRISON HEALTH CARE?

Most of our examples of the problems presented by prison health care and the means of solving them have come from our experience with the Massachusetts jails and prisons, visits to many others, and on site visits, standards meetings, and annual conferences of the National Commission. Massachusetts is by no means unique. What we have learned from our examinations of major issues in Massachusetts corrections can be applied to jails and prisons in county, state, and federal systems throughout the United States. Visits to jails in other states and in England confirm this. We can list the most important lessons:

1. Strong reformers, relying on the force of their personalities, can have profound effects on the prisons they direct, but the reforms do not outlast the reformers.
2. Reform by liberal-minded citizens, strengthened only by their resolve to change things, can raise the consciousness of the community temporarily, but cannot succeed without garnering support from the other parts of the community, which, it seems, would rather forget that prisons exist.
3. The courts, from the Supreme Court down, have taken a strong interest in protecting the civil rights of prison and jail inmates and have served admirably as overseers to guarantee the civil rights of inmates as well as other groups presently at risk.
4. Along with the courts, several professional societies interested in health issues have written and disseminated standards by which professional practice and facilities have been upgraded in U.S. jails and prisons. The nurses, who are on the front line of prison health care, were first to establish professional standards; law, corrections, and medicine followed.
5. Accreditation of jails and prisons works well, for the present, but standards are only the mechanism for stating the goals of an effort to improve prison medicine. If accreditation programs are not vigor-

ously promoted, the standards will be no more useful than all the other well-intentioned efforts of the last two centuries to improve prison conditions.

Written standards and accreditation programs based on them have an important advantage over other methods of reform, however. Standards are designed to reform the *system* by which medical care is given to prison inmates. Because they are formulated by a negotiation process of their own, and are not imposed by executive fiat or by dint of a strong reformer's will, standards are more likely to be successful in the long run.

Reforms in the system have prompted other changes in the ways medical care is provided. The major change, in accord with the tenor of the times, is to remove many of the responsibilities for health care from the public sector and contract them out to private, for-profit enterprises. The idea is attractive, but, as we have seen, in practice it is no panacea. Privatization is attractive because it effectively separates the caring from the custodial or penal functions of the jail. Doctors and nurses on contract to an outside firm are free to function as doctors and nurses. The unclear relationships between care and punishment are left to the contract negotiations and not to the day-to-day operation of the clinic. That is, in theory at least.

On the negative side, however, the privatization of prison health care is frankly motivated by the desire for private profits and public cost reductions. It remains an open question whether, in fact, this equation is anything more than rhetoric. It also remains an open question, even if private profits and public savings are possible, whether other social costs might yet make privatization unworkable or, at least, undesirable. If, for instance, the economics of privatization depends on full jails, the profit motive may favor incarceration over alternative sentencing methods.

We noted on table 1, above, just how little attention has been paid to the prison health problem. Jail suicide is a major problem and yet of the 2,919 scientific articles on suicide in the professional literature, only thirty-three articles deal specifically with prison suicide. Of the 369 articles on rape, only five deal with prison rape. Of the 6,013 articles on cirrhosis of the liver, a common consequence of alcohol abuse, only one article deals specifically with cirrhosis among the prison population. Of the 11,393 articles on hepatitis, commonly associated with homosexual activity and abuse of injected drugs, only seventeen articles deal specifically with hepatitis among prisoners, common victims of the disease. Homosexuality, although it is not a disease, is another major health issue in jails and prisons; yet of the 1,578 articles appearing in the scientific literature, only fourteen deal specifically with homosexuality and prison. Finally, of the 7,069 articles on trauma, certainly a major problem in jails and prisons, only eleven deal specifically with trauma among the imprisoned population. AIDS occurs among prisoners, especially in the New York City area, far more commonly than outside, yet no significant medical literature deals with AIDS in prisons.

One important point has been learned only imperfectly: lasting changes cannot be made in the correctional system and, specifically, in the prison medical system, until we know more about these systems. Careful research on the prison population, their physical and mental makeup, the nature of the ailments seen in prisons, the ways of treating them, and investigations of how jails and prisons work, management studies of how prisons are governed, and more are absolutely necessary. To date, we have seen very few carefully designed studies. Too many have been based on quick surveys or, worse yet, incompletely sampled questionnaires. In place of careful studies, we have anecdote, conjecture, and prejudgment. There are too few scientific studies of the major medical problems found among prison inmates to allow us to make informed decisions about medical practice or health policy.

WHAT IS DIFFERENT ABOUT PRISON MEDICINE?

To understand prison health care we must understand that the prison population is a biased sample of the general population and that the prison is a unique environment for the practice of medicine. The failure to appreciate or accept how different prison medicine is from the rest of medicine has interfered with establishing lasting, workable, and effective health care systems in prisons.

The overwhelming maleness, the preponderance of dyslexia, peptic ulcer, violent aggressive behavior, epilepsy, alcohol and drug abuse and addiction, possible excesses of male hormones, along with a notably low incidence of hypertension reinforce the view that we need to learn a great deal more about the biology of chronic criminal offenders. This is not to say, as some authors have maintained, that there is a criminal type or that most crime is biologically motivated. However, there is almost certainly something important to be learned from careful study of the biology of the recidivist offender.

The prisons themselves are a strange environment for physicians, nurses, and other health care providers. Health professionals are not prepared intellectually or emotionally for the vicissitudes of working in such an antitherapeutic environment. Moreover, health professionals usually do not get the emotional or even financial support they need to survive in such a place. Imprisonment colors every action and idea of both the prisoners and the men and women who look after them. The apparent incongruities, ironies, and administrative difficulties of having the same institution responsible for the care and punishment of convicted felons implies that we need to learn a great deal more about the attitudes and motives on which "correctional" (or are they penal?) policies are based.

Finally, there are immense and complex questions about the proper use of prisons in the first place. Jurists, philosophers, criminologists, and politicians must thrash out anew for each generation theories of crime and ways of dealing with it. At present, so great have been medical advances in understanding other areas of human life, that what we might call "the medicalization of crime" has been offered as a possible approach to providing a rationale for prison programs.

Psychopharmacologists have developed many powerful drugs to alter mood and control behavior. Psychoendocrinologists are learning much about how shifting hormones, naturally or therapeutically, profoundly affect emotions and actions. *If* criminal behavior, and this is a big assumption yet to be adequately tested, is *primarily* biologically motivated, then drugs, surgery, and other medical interventions would be appropriate. The idea is attractive because it promises scientific control where moral, social, and psychological efforts have failed.

We can only take an agnostic position on this important question: we do not know. It would be nice if it were true. Diseases once attributed to possession by demons are now treated with psychotherapy and psychotropic drugs. Perhaps in the future, when we know more about the relationships between mind, body, and behavior, we will be able to treat criminal behaviors, too, but we cannot agree on the extent to which we have a right to control or alter prisoners. For now, the human animal remains far too complex for us to prescribe such simple remedies for the social, psychological, and biological disorders labeled criminal behavior.

In *Care and Punishment*, we have not been interested primarily in the large philosophical issues. Our interest has been practical. Crimes will be committed; criminals will be incarcerated; and while in jails and prisons, prisoners will often get sick or will suffer exacerbations of illnesses they already had when they entered jail. Because the state, municipality, or federal government assumes responsibility for the welfare of the inmates whose personal liberty they have taken away, representatives of the government are obligated to provide or find adequate medical care.

Despite the magnitude and complexity of the problem, prisons and prisoners (not to mention crime and correction) have not been studied with anything even approaching the rigor of scientific method. It would be a good idea, indeed, to bring research into prisons so that finally accurate and reliable data could replace anecdote. Only then will there be a rational approach to prison management and, in time, an effective means of dealing with criminal behavior.

Men and women who work in prisons—superintendents, guards, health care personnel—and the inmates who live in prisons are probably right in saying that only those who have been there can really know what they are like. We do not dispute this statement although these people often have intensely subjective opinions; but the fact remains that we can no longer have two worlds, that behind the wall and that in front of the wall, with little communication. The courts have required that the standards of decency and medical care established for the community-at-large must hold for the imprisoned. Prisons cost money to build and to run. Until recently, that money came from the public coffers exclusively. As long as jails and prisons are run by public money, policy makers outside the walls must have easy understanding of the needs inside. For all these reasons, we must dispel the myth that only the men and women who have had firsthand knowledge of life in the jails and prisons can even imagine what it must be like and that only they should make the rules.

CONCLUSION

Lacking a sense of history, prison administrators and social reformers are condemned to repeat the policies of the past as if they were new. Social trends, intellectual fashions, religious influences, scientific theories all come and go, but they do not disappear forever or entirely. A perfect example is that of managed care in the jails and prisons run as profit-making enterprises. This was the principal method of running a jail in colonial times in the New World. Once again, the country is in eager pursuit of ways to minimize the role of central government and, in the interests of cutting public expenditures, has been attracted to the idea of letting private, for-profit companies build, staff, and run prisons.

The most successful prisons and jails are run with a clear understanding of how they differ from other social institutions. The most effective health professionals working within these unique institutions are sensitive to the conflicting goals of care and punishment. The profit motive may not be the most engaging social force for reforming correctional institutions and medical services within them, but at least a businesslike approach *can* introduce careful analysis where in the past sentiment reigned supreme. The suffering of the imprisoned (and of their keepers) has obscured the effectiveness of a rational management plan.

Assuming that there is sufficient money to allow the system to work, acceptance of the published standards, rigorous oversight of adherence to the standards by agencies outside the departments of correction, and professional pride in work well done will do more to assure the constitutionally mandated rights of prisoners to medical care than any amount of well-intentioned arm waving and finger pointing.

The human political animal being what he is, it will always be easier to find scapegoats than to face squarely the deficiencies of the jail health system. If we really want to help, there are practical and effective measures we can take, but first we must ask ourselves, individually and collectively, whether we want to. For until we have agreed on what we expect jails and prisons to accomplish for the welfare of the prisoner and the good of society, we will continue to vacillate between care and punishment.

NOTES
SELECTED BIBLIOGRAPHY
INDEX

Notes

CHAPTER 1. THE CULT OF PERSONALITY IN PRISON REFORM

1. A history of the Norfolk Prison Colony was written by an admiring student of Howard Gill's, Thomas Yakhub. We thank Howard Gill for sharing with us a typescript of Thomas Yakhub's history, dated 15 January 1936. This history was eventually reprinted in *A Report on the Development of Penological Treatment at Norfolk Prison Colony in Massachusetts*, ed. Carl R. Doering (New York: Bureau of Social Hygiene, Inc., 1940). We acknowledge our debt to this fascinating document, citing it as "Doering" in the text.

2. "The Van Waters Case, Including the Full Text of the Decision of the Impartial [*sic*] Commission," pamphlet published by the Friends of Framingham, 1949. The fifteen-page pamphlet sold for ten cents. See also J. B. Rowley, *The Lady in Box 99: The Story of Miriam Van Waters* (Greenwich, Conn.: Seabury Press, 1962).

3. Direct quotations of Howard Gill's comments throughout this chapter are drawn from tapes of the authors' interviews with Howard Gill conducted in June 1985. They are hitherto unpublished.

4. The Norfolk Prison Colony has been described in a pamphlet apparently written by members of the Norfolk Colony staff and dated 30 November 1932. Because it captures the flavor as well as the facts of the Norfolk Colony story, we quote from it extensively.

CHAPTER 2. THE PRISON HEALTH PROJECT

1. "Report of the Medical Advisory Committee on State Prisons to the Commissioner of Correction and the Secretary of Human Services of the Commonwealth of Massachusetts," Massachusetts Department of Correction, publication #6109, 29 December 1971. We refer to this important document as the "Madoff Report" in recognition of the committee chairman, Morton Madoff.

CHAPTER 3. THE JUDICIAL APPROACH

1. Profit is clearly not the chief motive in defending prisoners' rights. Several law firms have discovered that prison inmates are slow to pay and, when they do pay at all, they are usually unable to pay the full fee. The Boston firm that handled the class action suit at Walpole, for example, began work on the case in 1977 and still had not received a cent for its work more than nine years later. Nonetheless, the firm has recently submitted its bill for handling the Walpole case—$750,000.

2. At the urging of the aggrieved citizens of the semirural town of Walpole, Massachusetts, MCI Walpole is now officially called Cedar Junction, but by all but the most enthusiastic public relations interests, the prison is still called Walpole.

3. Material quoted in this chapter was drawn from interviews with Scott Lewis and Alfred DiSimone. All interpretations and conclusions are those of the authors.

Selected Bibliography

BOOKS

American Bar Association. *Medical and Health Care in Jails, Prisons, and Other Correctional Facilities*. Washington, D.C.: American Bar Association in conjunction with the American Medical Association, 1973.

American Correctional Association. *Manual of Standards for Adult Correctional Institutions*. Rockville, Md.: American Correctional Association, 1977.

American Psychiatric Association. *Diagnostic and Statistical Manual of Mental Disorders*, 2d and 3d eds. (*DSM-II* and *DSM-III*). Washington, D.C., American Psychiatric Association, 1968, 1980.

Brecher, E. M., and R. D. DellaPenna. *Prescriptive Package: Health Care in Correctional Institutions*. National Institute of Law Enforcement and Criminal Justice. Washington, D.C.: GPO, 1975.

The Captive Patient. Report of the Kentucky Public Health Association, 1974.

Cheever, John. *Falconer*. New York: Knopf, 1975.

Cleckley, H. *The Mask of Sanity*. St. Louis: C.V. Mosby, 1964.

Cohen, S., and L. Taylor. *Psychological Survival*. New York: Pantheon, 1972.

Cormier, B. M. *The Watcher and the Watched*. Montreal: Tundra, 1975.

Danto, B. L. *Jail House Blues*. Orchard Lake, Mich.: Epic Publications, 1973.

Doering, Carl R., ed. *A Report on the Development of Penological Treatment at Norfolk Prison Colony in Massachusetts*. New York: Bureau of Social Hygiene, 1940.

Derro, R. A. *Admission Health Evaluations of Inmates of a City-County Workhouse*. Report by St. Paul-Ramsey Hospital Medical Education and Research Foundation, 1976.

Dobash, R. *The Imprisonment of Women*. London: Blackwell, 1986.

Eyeman, J. S. *Prisons for Women*. Springfield, Ill.: C.C. Thomas, 1971.

Foucault, M. *Discipline and Punish: The Birth of the Prison*. Trans. A. Sheridan. New York: Pantheon, 1977.

Giallombardo, Rose. *Society of Women: A Study of a Women's Prison*. New York: John Wiley, 1966.

264 † SELECTED BIBLIOGRAPHY

Glueck, S., and E. Glueck. *Juvenile Delinquents Grown Up.* New York: Commonwealth Fund, 1940.
Goffman, E. *Asylums.* Garden City, N.Y.: Anchor, 1961.
Goldsmith, S. B. *Prison Health: Travesty of Justice.* New York: PRODIST, 1974.
Gunn, J., and D. P. Farrington. *Abnormal Offenders, Delinquency, and the Criminal Justice System.* Current Research in Forensic Psychiatry and Psychology. New York: Wiley, 1982.
Guze, S. B. *Criminality and Psychiatric Disorders.* New York: Oxford University Press, 1976.
Hall, E. T. *The Hidden Dimension.* New York: Doubleday, 1966.
Hammett, T. M. *AIDS in Correctional Facilities: Issues and Options.* Rockville, Md.: U.S. Department of Justice, National Institute of Justice, 1986.
Hawkins, G. *The Prison: Policy and Practice.* Chicago: University of Chicago Press, 1976.
Ignatieff, M. *A Just Measure of Pain: The Penitentiary in the Industrial Revolution, 1750–1850.* New York: Pantheon, 1978.
Jamieson, K. M., and T. J. Flanagan, eds. *Sourcebook of Criminal Justice Statistics—1986.* U.S. Department of Justice, Bureau of Justice Statistics. Washington, D.C.: GPO, 1987.
Jervis, N. *Prison Health Reform: Four Case Studies.* New York: Health Policy Advisory Center, 1975.
Johnston, N. *The Human Cage: A Brief History of Prison Architecture.* Philadelphia: Walker, 1973.
Jurczak, D. M. *The Correctional Psychiatrist in the Federal Prison System.* Danbury, Conn.: Federal Correctional Institution at Danbury, n.d.
Kobler, A., and E. Stotland. *The End of Hope.* Philadelphia: Free Press, 1964.
Mack, J. E., ed. *Borderline States in Psychiatry.* New York: Grune and Stratton, 1975.
Maestro, M. *Cesare Beccaria and the Origins of Penal Reform.* Philadelphia: Temple University Press, 1973.
Mark, V. H., and F. R. Ervin. *Violence and the Brain.* New York: Harper and Row, 1970.
Menninger, K. *The Crime of Punishment.* New York: Viking, 1968.
Mullen, J., K. J. Chabotar, and D. M. Carrow. *The Privatization of Corrections.* U.S. Department of Justice, National Institute of Justice, February 1985.
Nagel, W. G. *The New Red Barn: A Critical Look at the Modern American Prison.* Philadelphia: Walker, 1973.
National Commission on Correctional Health Care. *Standards for Health Services in Jails, 1987.* Chicago: NCCHC, 1987.
National Commission on Correctional Health Care. *Standards for Health Services in Juvenile Detention Facilities, 1987.* Chicago: NCCHC, 1987.
National Commission on Correctional Health Care. *Standards for Health Services in Prisons, 1987.* Chicago, NCCHC, 1987.
Novick, L. F., and M. S. Al-Ibrahim. *Health Problems in the Prison Setting: A Clinical and Administrative Approach.* Springfield, Ill.: C.C. Thomas, 1977.

Ostfeld, A. *Stress, Crowding, and Blood Pressure in Prison.* New York: Erlbaum Associates, 1987.

Prout, C. *Prison Health Project: Final Report.* Boston: Massachusetts Health Research Institute, 1974.

Rothman, D. J. *The Discovery of the Asylum.* Boston: Little, Brown, 1971.

Rowley, J. B. *The Lady in Box 99: The Story of Miriam Van Waters.* Greenwich, Conn.: Seabury, 1962.

Smith, R. *Prison Health Care.* London: Taylor and Francis, 1984.

United Nations. *Standard Minimum Rules for the Treatment of Prisoners.* Resolution adopted 30 August 1955 by the First United Nations Congress on the Prevention of Crime and the Treatment of Offenders.

Wilson, J. Q., Herrnstein, R. J. *Crime and Human Nature: The Definitive Study of the Causes of Crime.* New York: Simon and Schuster, 1985.

Wooden, W. S., and J. Parker. *Men Behind Bars: Sexual Exploitation in Prison.* New York: Plenum, 1982.

ARTICLES AND PAMPHLETS

Alston et al. v. *Hogan et al.* U.S. District Court, Civil Action No. 77-3519-G.

"Annual Report of the Superintendent of MCI Concord." Massachusetts Department of Correction. Boston, 1937.

"Annual Report of the Superintendent of MCI Norfolk." Massachusetts Department of Correction. Boston, 1937.

Bach-y-Rita, G., J. R. Lion, C. E. Climent, and F. R. Ervin. "Episodic Dyscontrol." *American Journal of Psychiatry* 127 (1971): 1473–78.

Bassuk, E. L., L. Rubin, and A. Lauriat. "Back to Bedlam: Are Shelters Becoming Alternative Institutions?" Harvard Medical School Department of Psychiatry, 1985, unpublished.

Blumstein, A., and J. Cohen. "Characterizing Criminal Careers." *Science* 237 (1987): 985–91.

Butler Committee. "Secure Hospital Units." *British Medical Journal* 5925 (1974): 215–16.

Carney, F. J. "Evaluation of Psychotherapy in a Maximum Security Prison." *Seminars in Psychiatry* 3 (1971): 363–75.

Chombard de Lauwe, P. "Famille et Habitation." Paris: Editions du Centre National de la Recherche Scientifique, 1959.

Christie, N. "Medical Care of Prisoners and Detainees." Presented at the CIBA Symposium on Medical Care of Prisoners and Detainees, 1973.

CIBA Foundation Symposium 16. *Medical Care of Prisoners and Detainees.* Amsterdam: Associated Scientific Publishers, 1973.

Culpepper, L., and J. Fromm. "Incarceration and Blood Pressure." Social Science Medicine 14 (1980): 571–74.

Curran, W. J. "Confidentiality and the Prediction of Dangerousness in Psychiatry." *New England Journal of Medicine* 293 (1975): 285–86.

266 † SELECTED BIBLIOGRAPHY

Curran, W. J., and W. Casscells. "Ethics in Human Experimentation Defined by National Commission." *New England Journal of Medicine* 296 (1977): 44–45.

Daniel, A. E., P. W. Harris, and S. A. Husain. "Differences Between Midlife Female Offenders and Those Less than 40." *American Journal of Psychiatry* 138 (1981): 1225–28.

D'Atri, D. A. "Crowding in Prison: The Relationship Between Changes in Housing Mode and Blood Pressure." *Psychosomatic Medicine* 43 (1981): 95–105.

Dubler, N. "Legal Issues in Corrections." Proceedings of the Third National Conference on Medical Care and Health Services in Correctional Institutions, Chicago. American Medical Association, 1979: 67–73.

Fitzgerald, W. J. "Health Problems in a Cohort of Prisoners at Intake and During Incarceration." *Journal of Prison and Jail Health* 4 (1984): 61–76.

Gaunay, W., and R. L. Gido. "Acquired Immune Deficiency Syndrome: A Demographic Profile of New York State Inmate Mortalities, 1981–1985." New York: N.Y. State Commission of Correction, 1986.

Goldsmith, S. B. "The Status of Prison Health Care." *Public Health Reports* 89 (1974): 569–75.

Gunn, J. "Social Factors and Epileptics in Prisons." *British Journal of Psychiatry* 124 (1974): 509–17.

Gunn, J., and G. Fenlon. "Epilepsy in Prisons: A Diagnostic Survey." *British Medical Journal* 4 (1969): 326–28.

Gunn, J., and J. Bonn. "Criminality and Violence in Epileptic Prisoners." *British Journal of Psychiatry* 118 (1971): 337–43.

Heller, M. S. "The Private Reflections of a Prison Psychiatrist." *Prison Journal* 54 (Autumn 1974): 15–33.

Kennedy, S. A. "A View from Inside." *American Journal of Nursing* 75 (1975): 417–20.

King, L. N., and S. Whitman. "Morbidity and Mortality Among Prisoners: An Epidemiologic Review." *Journal of Prison Health* 1 (1981): 7–29.

King, L., R. Reynolds, and A. Young. "Utilization of Former Military Medical Corpsmen in the Provision of Jail Health Services." *American Journal of Public Health* 67 (1977): 730–34.

Lewis, D. O., J. H. Pincus, S. S. Shano, and G. H. Glaser. "Psychomotor Epilepsy and Violence in a Group of Incarcerated Adolescent Boys." *American Journal of Psychiatry* 139 (1982): 882–87.

London, W. P., and B. M. Taylor. "Bipolar Disorders in a Forensic Setting." *Comprehensive Psychiatry* 23 (1982): 33–37.

McLean, E. K. "Prison as Humanity." *Lancet* 1 (1975): 507–11.

Madoff Report. See "Report of the Medical Advisory Committee on [Massachusetts] State Prisons."

Meehl, I. Q. "A Psychosocial Description of Penitentiary Inmates." *Archives of General Psychiatry* 29 (1973): 663–67.

Mills, M., and N. Morris. "Prisoners as Laboratory Animals." *Society* 1073 (1974): 64–66.

Mindlin, R. L., and L. Pollack. "Comprehensive Medical Examinations at the Charles Street Jail." Privately circulated report, 1973.
Moore, M. "Forced Feeding of Prisoners." *Lancet* 1 (1974): 1109.
Morris, A. "Extending Public Understanding of Crime and Its Treatment." Correctional Research Bulletin no. 23: 1–28. Boston; Massachusetts Correctional Association, 1973.
National Commission on Correctional Health Care. Proceedings of the National Conferences on Correctional Health Care, Chicago, 1979, 1981.
"The New Prison at Norfolk, Massachusetts," pamphlet apparently written by the Norfolk Colony staff, 30 November 1932.
Novick, L. F., R. DellaPenna, M. S. Schwartz, and R. Lowenstein. "Health Status of the New York City Prison Population." Presented at the 103d annual meeting of the American Public Health Association, Epidemiology Section, November 1975.
Parkhurst, L. "Report of the Special Commission on the Advisability of Providing Additional Penal Institutions and Equipment." H. Rept. 2087. Massachusetts Legislative Documents, Boston, 1939.
Prout, C. "Prison Health Services." *New England Journal of Medicine* 290 (1974): 856–57.
"Report of the Medical Advisory Committee on State Prisons to the Commissioner of Correction and the Secretary of Human Services of the Commonwealth of Massachusetts," Massachusetts Department of Correction, publication no. 6109, 29 December 1971. [Madoff Report]
Rosenfeld, E. D. "An Evaluation of Medical and Health Care Services at the Attica Correctional Facility." New York: Rosenfeld Associates, 1972.
Rosenhahn, S. L. "On Being Sane in Insane Places." *Science* 179 (1973): 250–58.
Salley, R. D., R. Khanna, W. Byrum, and L. D. Hutt. "REM Sleep and EEG Abnormalities in Criminal Psychopaths." *Perceptual and Motor Skills* 51 (1981): 715–22.
"Standards for Services in Prisons." Chicago: National Commission of Correctional Health Care, 1987.
Twaddle, A. C. "Utilization of Physician Services by a Captive Population: An Analysis of Sick Call in a State Prison." *Journal of Health and Social Behavior* 17 (1976): 236–48.
"The Van Waters Case, Including the Full Text of the Decision of the Impartial [*sic*] Commission." Friends of Framingham, 1949, pamphlet.
Whalen, R. P., and J.J.A. Lyons. "Medical Problems of 500 Prisoners on Admission to a County Jail." *Public Health Reports* 77 (1962): 497–502.
Yeudall, L. T., D. Fromm-Auch, and P. Davies. "Neuropsychological Impairment of Persistent Delinquency." *Journal of Nervous and Mental Disease* 170 (1982): 257–65.

Index

Accreditation, of prison health care systems, 121, 235, 240–47
Adorno, Eli, 190
AIDS, 13, 186–92; and condoms, 190; and education, 189; and Kaposi's sarcoma, 188; testing for, 188; treatment of, 189
Alcohol abuse. *See* Substance abuse
Alcoholics Anonymous, 197
American Academy of Physicians for the Incarcerated, 128
American Bar Association (ABA), 4, 89, 144, 233
American College of Surgeons, 34, 38
American Correctional Association (ACA), 4, 131, 190, 233, 239
American Federation of State, County, and Municipal Employees (AFSCME), 128
American Medical Association (AMA), 4, 87, 89, 233, 240
American Nursing Association (ANA), 4, 155, 233
American Psychiatric Association (APA), 184, 210–11
American Public Health Association (APHA), 4, 73
Amphetamines, 202–03
Amytal, 202
Anesthesia, 173
Angel dust (PCP), 198, 218

Anger: of guards, 153; of inmates, 59, 95, 139, 143, 147, 221; of physicians, 9, 59, 68
Antisocial behavior, 137, 210–12
Attica State Prison (N.Y.), 3, 43, 130

Backman, Jack, 96
Barbituates, 202
Barton, Clara, 40
Bates, Sanford, 26, 30, 35, 93
Baumgartner, Leona, 56
Beccaria, Cesare Bonesana, 230
Bentham, Jeremy, 116
Bicknell, William, 51, 55, 61
Blodgett, James T., 8, 9
Bloomberg, Wilfred, 34, 37–39
Body cavity searches, 14, 140
Boone, John O., 52, 61, 95
Borderline personality disorder, 210–12
Boston City Hospital, 67, 69, 71
Bridgewater State Hospital and Prison (MCI Bridgewater; Mass.), 39, 40, 60, 69, 84–85
Broadmoor Hospital (Great Britain), 171
Bulfinch, Charles, 142
Bunte, Doris, 96
Burger, Warren, 116
Butler Committee, 171

Psychoendocrinology, 255–56
Psychopharmacology, 255–56
Psychosis, and criminal behavior, 171, 215
Psychosurgery, 207–08
Punishment, definition of, 150, 205, 228

Quaalude, 203

Radiologists, 175
Rage, 207, 213
Rape, 172–73, 184–85, 190
Rappaport, Allan H., 126
Recidivism, 10, 57, 171, 210, 225
Reform: of prison health care, 3–6, 9, 42–43, 64, 87–90, 104–09, 111–13, 114–16; of prisons, 3–6, 9–10, 21–25, 34–35, 40–41, 248–49, 252–53. *See also* Norfolk Prison Colony; Prison Health Project
Rehabilitation, and prison health care, 35–41, 46–51, 53, 233
Richard, Ray, 95
Rights, of prisoners, 47–49, 88–90, 100, 145–46, 161, 189, 227–38, 262*n*
Rikers Island Prison (N.Y.), 99, 140, 174, 186
Robert Wood Johnson Foundation, 71
Robinson, Margaret (Sunny), 55–56, 80
Rockefeller Foundation, 21, 35, 75
Rosenbloom, Joseph, 96
Rowan, Joseph, 150
Rundles, Frank, 56

Sargent, Francis W., 51–53, 60
Scherl, Donald, 86
Seconal, 202
Security, in prisons, 123–24, 139, 141, 144, 146, 151–53, 158–60, 164–66, 168–69, 171–73, 189, 193, 216
Sexual behavior, in prison, 40, 183–86, 191–92, 218
Sexual offenders, 60, 172–73, 218

Shattuck Hospital (Mass.), 61, 66
Shaw, George Bernard, 208
Sheraton syndrome, 132
Shirley Prerelease Center, 52, 55, 83
Shirley Youth Services Correctional Facility (Industrial Home for Boys), 52, 55
Sick call, 130, 160–61, 179
Sieracki, Louis, 34
Silva, Dr. (physician-inmate, Norfolk Prison Colony), 38–39
Silverdale Detention Center (Tenn.), 118, 120
Smith v. *Wade*, 239
Solitary confinement, 148–50, 161
Sopor, 203
Specter, Arlen, 114
Speed, 202–03
Standards, for prison health care, 87–88, 119, 131–34, 227–49
Starrett, Barbara, 99
Stimulants, 162, 202
Substance abuse, 194–205; and AIDS, 186; alcohol, 141, 170, 194–97, 204; cocaine, 198; and criminal behavior, 60, 139, 141, 170, 176; Darvon-N, 201, 203; and detoxification, 53–55, 57–58, 83, 199–203; illicit drug traffic, 163, 166, 194; heroin, 198–200, 204; and medical records, 176, Narcan, 199; opium, 201; and rehabilitation, 53–55, 57–58, 196; Talwin, 75–76, 203; testing for, 175, 199; and theft of drugs, 163; treatment programs for, 53–55, 57–58, 83, 199–203; withdrawal from, 177, 195, 196–97, 200–03
Suffolk County House of Correction (Deer Island; Mass.), 223
Suffolk County Jail (Charles Street Jail; Boston), 74, 141, 142, 242
Suicide, 40–41, 137, 150, 220–22
Surgery, in prison, 173–74
Syphilis, 191, 224

CONTEMPORARY COMMUNITY HEALTH SERIES